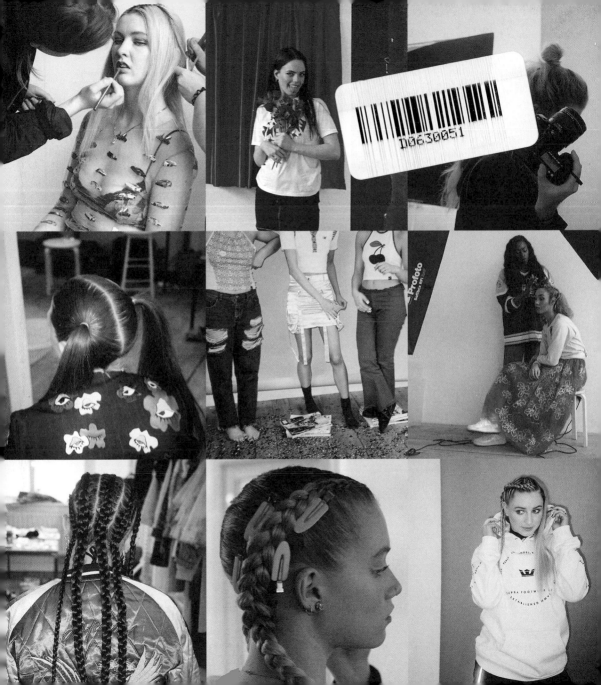

D0830051

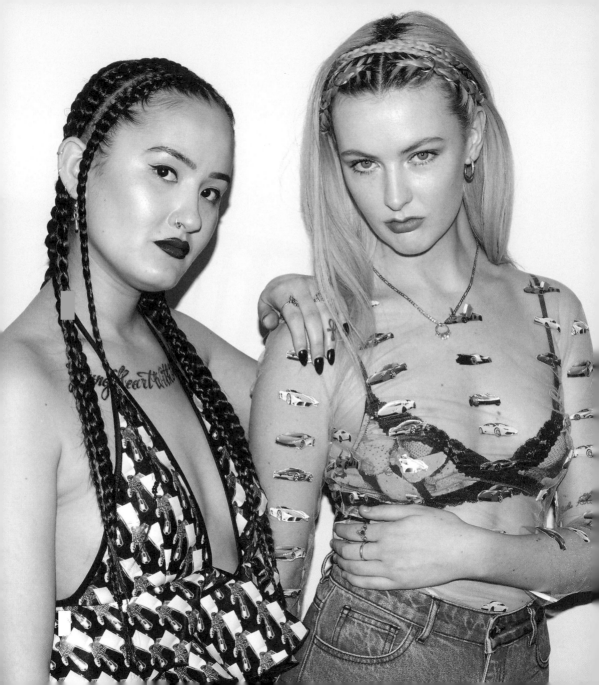

BY
JESSY
LINTON
&
TAIBA
AKHUETIE

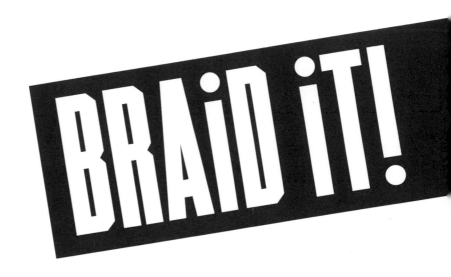

Photography by Olivia Richardson

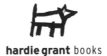

hardie grant books

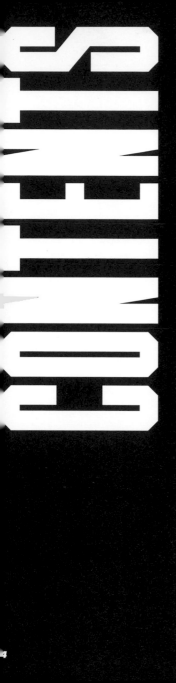

CONTENTS

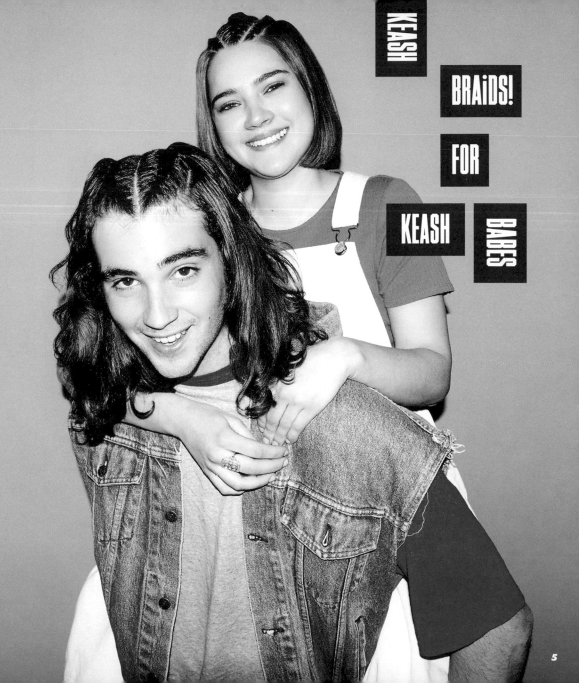

KEASH

BRAiDS!

FOR

KEASH BABES

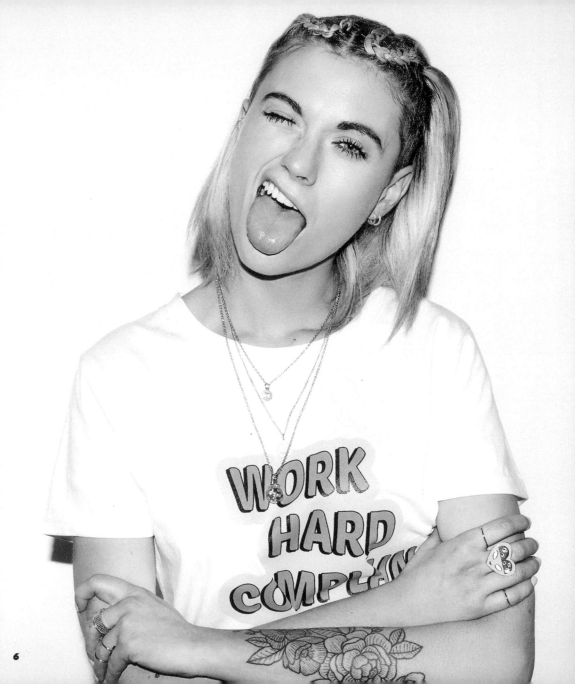

Welcome to your definitive guide to hair braiding from the girls at Keash Braids.

Long hair, strong hair, weak hair, short hair, thick hair, curly hair, afro hair; shoulder-length or past-your-bum; up in a top-knot or tucked behind your ears – whatever you do with your 'do' and however you wear it, there's something in here for you.

With more than 30 styles on 30 real girls (they're all our mates), this is the authentic DIY guide to getting your hair perfectly plaited at home. From classic cornrows to twisted buns, rainbow roots to punk braids, we talk you through our cult styles in an easy step-by-step approach. Jam-packed with original tricks, tips and hacks to make your hair happy, this is every girl's braid bible. Keep it to hand at all times. Share it with your friends. Learn the styles, improve your skills, but most of all, enjoy yourself.

Note: Each tutorial has a key that recommends a technique to use from The Skills (pages 12–21) and suggests where you may need a friend to help achieve the style. This is only a guideline so feel free to try out, for example, French Braids where we recommend Dutch Braids, and if you're a competent braider don't shy away from attempting all the styles on yourself.

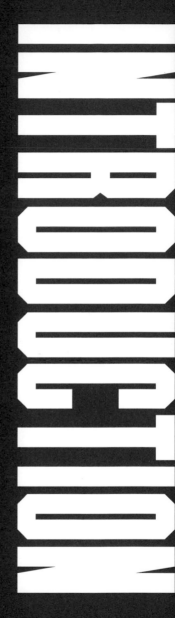

INTRODUCTION

Keash Braids was founded in the long, hot summer of 2014 by BFFs Taiba and Jessy. After a sticky London heatwave, they decided there had to be more to life than a scruffy ponytail.

It began like all great plans – with an Instagram account, which served as a simple braid appreciation page. Jessy and Taiba spent months driving their flatmates loopy with bobby pins and wigs, practising new styles and discovering new techniques, until everything suddenly snowballed and the two decided to start their own company, Keash Braids.

Taiba was already proficient with a pintail comb, having grown up with Nigerian parents and a mother well-practised in hair braiding, and Jessy's arts degree meant she was able to whip up a website in no time.

In March 2015, the pair set up (temporary) shop with their first pop-up salon in East London, which saw Instagram icons and TV presenters come through their sparkly doors. Mums and daughters, best mates, boys – everyone wanted a slice of the Keash pie. Since then, Taiba and Jessy have styled music videos and campaigns, held a residency at Urban Outfitters' flagship store on Oxford Street and braided more heads than they can count.

This is Keash Braids' first book – an homage to braids' heritage and a celebration of its fresh adoption into youth culture today.

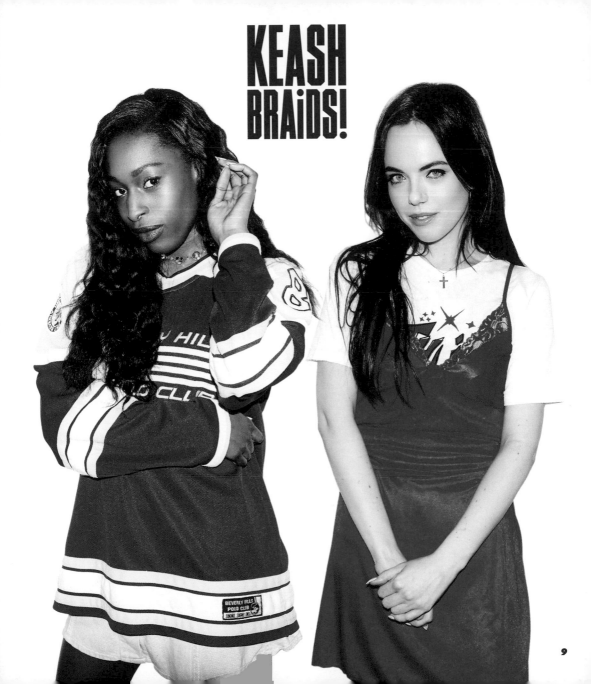

KEASH
BRAiDS!

TOOLS

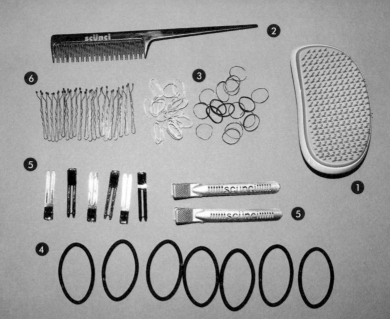

2 — scünci

6

3

5

1

4

PRODUCTS

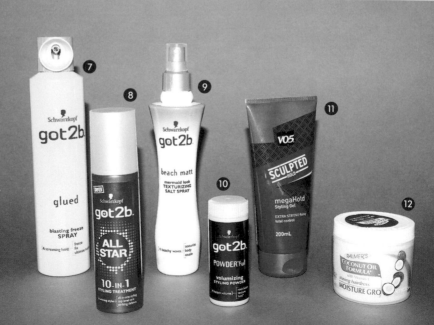

7 — Schwarzkopf got2b. glued
blasting freeze SPRAY

8 — Schwarzkopf got2b. ALL STAR 10-IN-1 STYLING TREATMENT

9 — Schwarzkopf got2b. beach matt mermaid look TEXTURIZING SALT SPRAY

10 — Schwarzkopf got2b. POWDER'ful volumizing STYLING POWDER

11 — VO5 SCULPTED HOLD megaHold Styling Gel EXTRA STRONG fixing total control 200mL

12 — PALMER'S COCONUT OIL FORMULA shining hairdress MOISTURE GRO

Let's get started! Here are the tools you will need in your basic braiding kit.

These styling tools will help you eager braiders to master some badass braids. Get to know your tools, practice your skills and before you know it you'll be a pro.

A pintail comb is an essential tool and will ensure perfect partings before you begin to braid. A clean, neat parting makes a huge difference to the final outcome of any style. Once the partings are in place use a Tangle Teezer (or any standard hairbrush) to brush and smooth the hair. If the hair is unbrushed and knotted it will be difficult to style, so make sure you prepare the hair properly.

Once the hair is parted and detangled, use a styling product to make the hair more manageable and easier to braid. Priming the hair with coconut oil is great for afro hair as it's oily and holds moisture, ideal for coarse hair. A lightweight styling cream (such as Got2B All Star Styling Treatment) works well on European hair as it makes the hair easier to work with and holds without looking greasy.

For those of you who want to achieve a more rough-and-ready, beachy look, add styling powder or dry shampoo to the roots before braiding the hair to add texture and volume. To really surf up the look use salt spray before styling to add body and a matte finish to the hair.

We use sectioning clips to keep partings in place while styling the hair to ensure you won't pick up hair from the wrong section.

Tie off the braids with polybands for a tidy finish. We use coloured loom bands when we are feeling thrifty and want to add a splash of colour to the style.

Last but not least, hairspray! It holds any style in place and controls flyaways, so always give your finished style a spritz.

What you need:

Tools:
1 Tangle Teezer
2 Scünci Pintail Comb
3 Scünci Black and Clear Polybands
4 Scünci Hair Bands
5 Scünci Sectioning Clips
6 Scünci Hair Grips

—

Products:
7 Got2B Glued Hairspray
8 Got2B All Star Styling Treatment (for European hair)
9 Got2B Salt Spray
10 Got2B Powder'ful Volumizing Styling Powder
11 V05 Mega Hold Gel
12 Palmer's Coconut Oil Hairdress (for coarse afro hair)

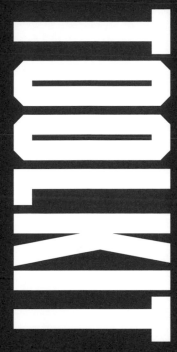

TOOLKIT

THE SKILLS

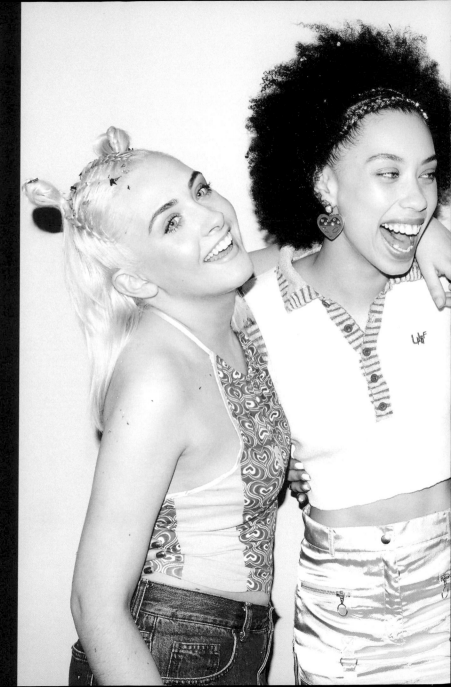

GET THE HANG OF THESE BASIC TECHNIQUES AND YOU'LL HAVE NO TROUBLE MAKING YOUR WAY THROUGH OUR HOW-TO HAIRDOS. REMEMBER: YOUR SKILLS WILL ONLY IMPROVE! PRACTICE MAKES PERFECT.

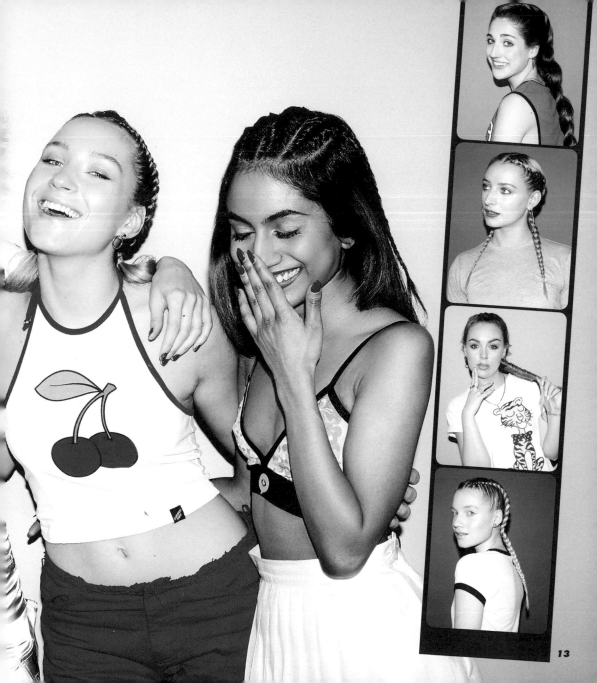

13

FRENCH BRAIDS

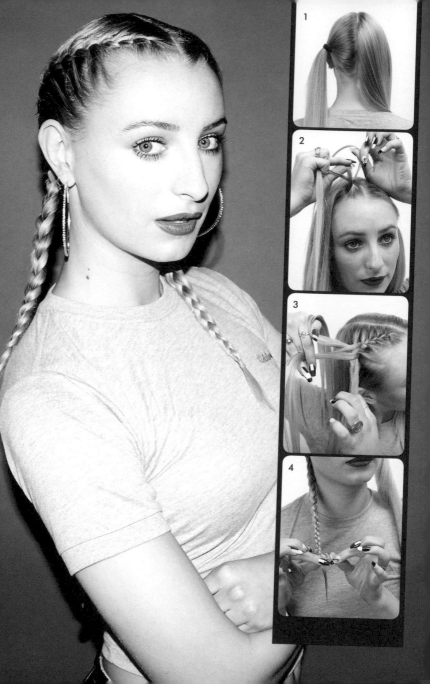

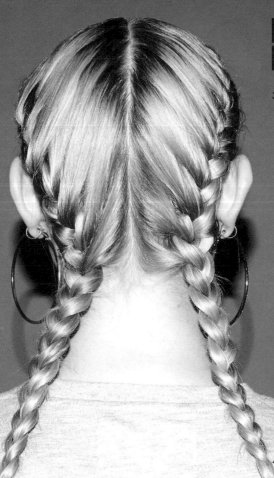

Step-by-step:

1 Begin with a centre
parting and continue the
parting down to the nape
of the neck, splitting the
hair into two even sections.
Tie off one section to keep
it out of the way and
smooth a styling product
(page 10) through the
loose side of hair to make
it more manageable.

2 Take a small section of
hair at the hairline and
split it into three strands.

   Tip: The smaller this
   section, the neater the
   braids will look!

   Begin by crossing the
   right strand over the
   middle strand and passing
   the middle strand to the
   right hand. Then cross the
   left strand over the new
   middle strand and pass
   the middle strand to the
   left hand.

   Note: If you're left-
   handed it may feel more
   comfortable to do this
   the opposite way round.

   Keep all three strands
   separate – you should
   always be holding one
   strand in the right hand
   and two strands in the
   left hand.

3 Using your right hand,
pick up a small section
of loose hair from the
right side and add it
to the right strand.
Cross the right strand
over the middle strand,
again keeping all strands
separate. Now, pass the
middle strand to your
right hand.

   Note: You should be
   holding one strand in
   your right hand and two
   strands in your
   left hand.

   Using your left hand,
   take a small section of
   loose hair from the left
   side and add it to the left
   strand. Cross the left
   strand over the middle
   strand and pass the
   middle strand to your
   left hand.

   Note: You should
   be holding one strand
   in your left hand and two
   strands in your right
   hand.

4 Continue the French
Braid by repeating step 3.
When you reach the nape
of the neck, continue with
a basic plait and tie off
at the ends of the hair.

   Let down the opposite
   side of hair and repeat
   the process to complete
   the style.

DUTCH BRAIDS

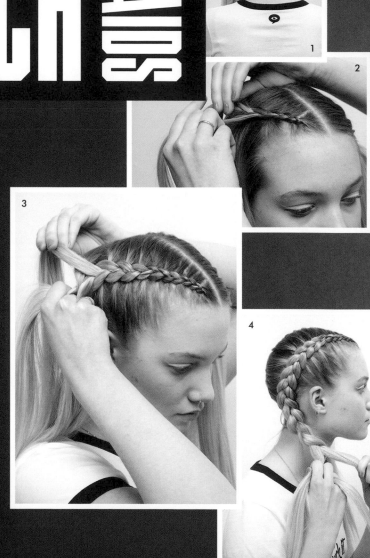

Step-by-step:

1   Begin with a centre parting and continue the parting down to the nape of the neck, splitting the hair into two even sections. Tie off one section to keep it out of the way and smooth a styling product (page 10) through the loose side of hair to make it more manageable.

2   Take a small section of hair at the hairline and split it into three strands.

    Tip: The smaller this section, the neater the braids will look!

    Begin by crossing the right strand under the middle strand and pass the middle strand to your right hand. Then cross the left strand under the new middle strand passing the middle strand to your left hand.

Note: If you're left-handed it may feel more comfortable to do this the other way round.

Keep all three strands separate – you should always be holding one strand in the right hand and two strands in the left hand.

3 Using your right hand, pick up a small section of loose hair from the right side and add it to the right strand. Cross the right strand under the middle strand, again keeping all strands separate. Now, pass the middle strand to your right hand. **Note:** You should be holding one strand in your right hand and two strands in your left hand.

Using your left hand, take a small section of loose hair from the left side and add it to the left strand.

Cross the left strand under the middle strand and pass the middle strand to your left hand.

Note: You should be holding one strand in your left hand and two strands in your right hand.

4 Continue the Dutch Braid by repeating step 3.

When you reach the nape of the neck, continue with a basic plait and tie off at the ends of the hair.

Let down the opposite side of hair and repeat the process to complete the style.

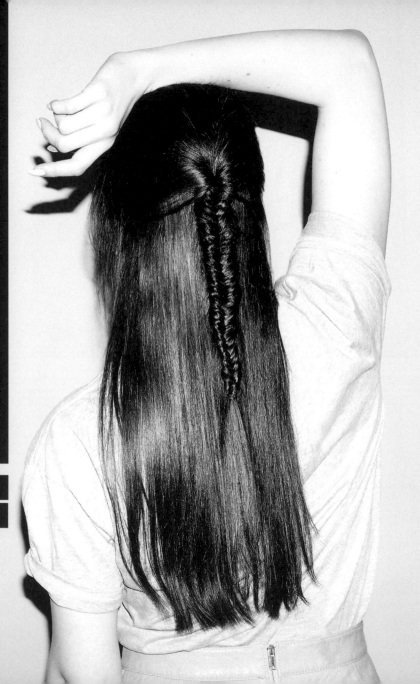

FISHTAIL PLAIT

SKILL LEVEL: EASY

NEED A FRIEND? NO!

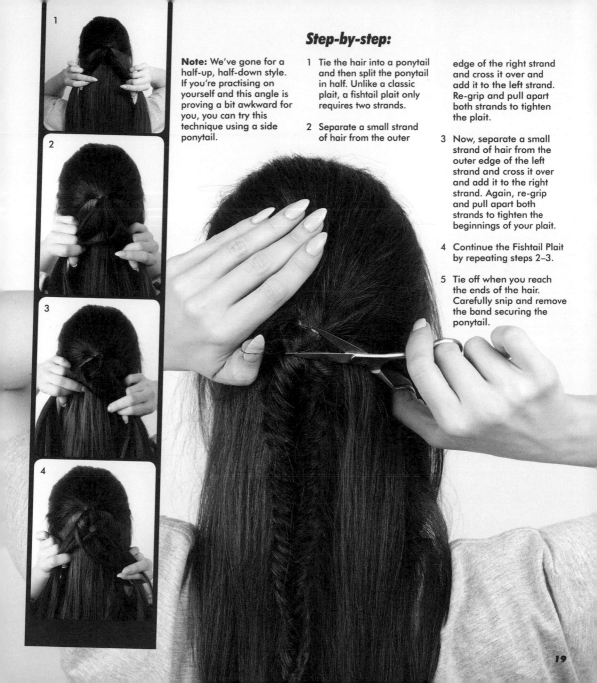

Step-by-step:

Note: We've gone for a half-up, half-down style. If you're practising on yourself and this angle is proving a bit awkward for you, you can try this technique using a side ponytail.

1 Tie the hair into a ponytail and then split the ponytail in half. Unlike a classic plait, a fishtail plait only requires two strands.

2 Separate a small strand of hair from the outer edge of the right strand and cross it over and add it to the left strand. Re-grip and pull apart both strands to tighten the plait.

3 Now, separate a small strand of hair from the outer edge of the left strand and cross it over and add it to the right strand. Again, re-grip and pull apart both strands to tighten the beginnings of your plait.

4 Continue the Fishtail Plait by repeating steps 2–3.

5 Tie off when you reach the ends of the hair. Carefully snip and remove the band securing the ponytail.

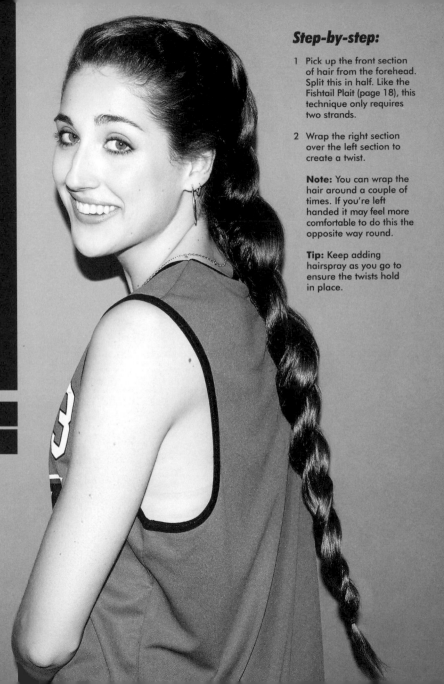

ROPE BRAID

SKILL LEVEL: EASY

NEED A FRIEND? NO!

Step-by-step:

1 Pick up the front section of hair from the forehead. Split this in half. Like the Fishtail Plait (page 18), this technique only requires two strands.

2 Wrap the right section over the left section to create a twist.

Note: You can wrap the hair around a couple of times. If you're left handed it may feel more comfortable to do this the opposite way round.

Tip: Keep adding hairspray as you go to ensure the twists hold in place.

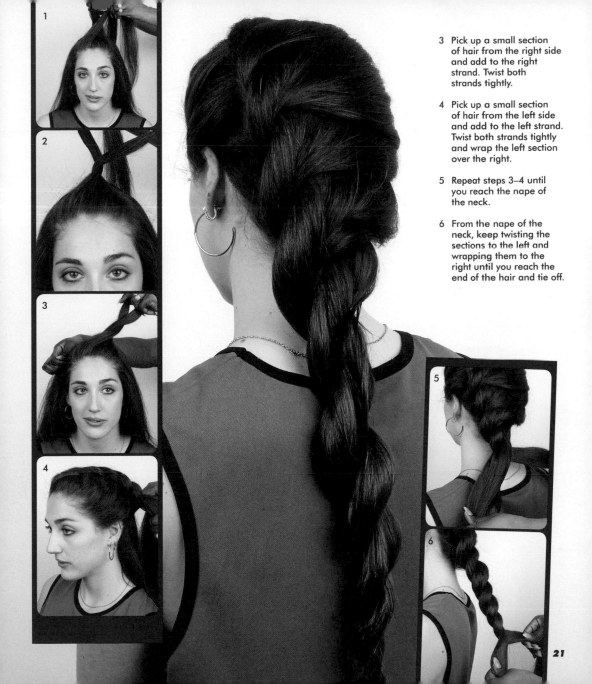

3 Pick up a small section of hair from the right side and add to the right strand. Twist both strands tightly.

4 Pick up a small section of hair from the left side and add to the left strand. Twist both strands tightly and wrap the left section over the right.

5 Repeat steps 3–4 until you reach the nape of the neck.

6 From the nape of the neck, keep twisting the sections to the left and wrapping them to the right until you reach the end of the hair and tie off.

21

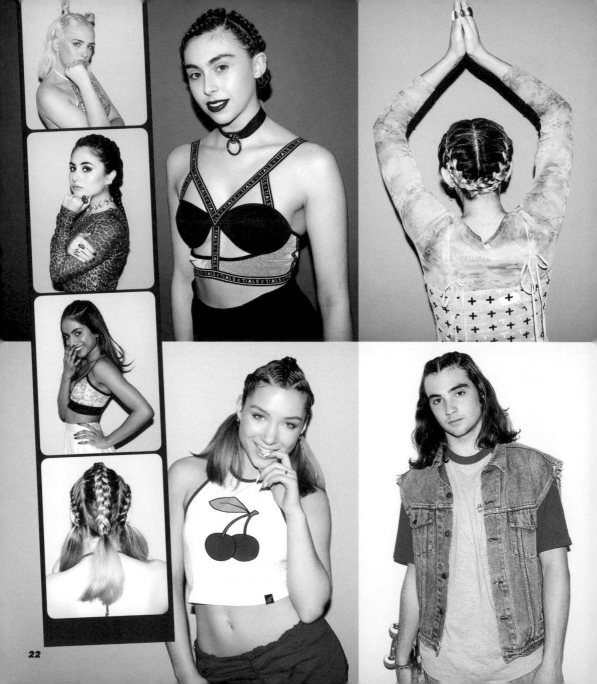

NOW YOU'VE FAMILIARISED YOURSELF WITH THE BASIC TECHNIQUES, IT'S TIME TO PUT THEM INTO PRACTICE. PLAY AROUND WITH PARTINGS, BE ADVENTUROUS AND TAKE THE TIME TO DEVELOP YOUR SKILLS AND STYLES.

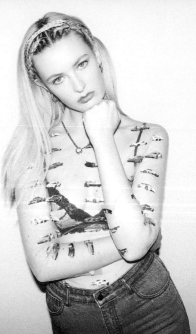

THE BRAIDS

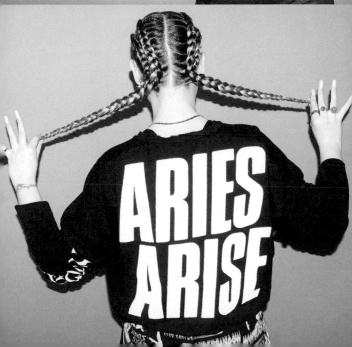

PART 1

PLAYGIRL BUNNY

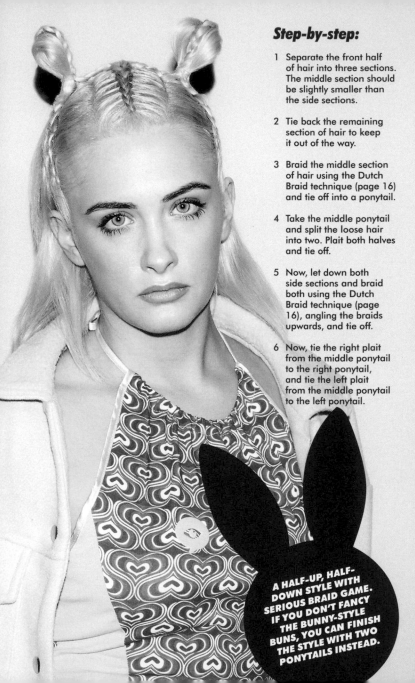

SKILL? *DUTCH BRAID*

NEED A FRIEND? *NO!*

Step-by-step:

1. Separate the front half of hair into three sections. The middle section should be slightly smaller than the side sections.

2. Tie back the remaining section of hair to keep it out of the way.

3. Braid the middle section of hair using the Dutch Braid technique (page 16) and tie off into a ponytail.

4. Take the middle ponytail and split the loose hair into two. Plait both halves and tie off.

5. Now, let down both side sections and braid both using the Dutch Braid technique (page 16), angling the braids upwards, and tie off.

6. Now, tie the right plait from the middle ponytail to the right ponytail, and tie the left plait from the middle ponytail to the left ponytail.

A HALF-UP, HALF-DOWN STYLE WITH SERIOUS BRAID GAME. IF YOU DON'T FANCY THE BUNNY-STYLE BUNS, YOU CAN FINISH THE STYLE WITH TWO PONYTAILS INSTEAD.

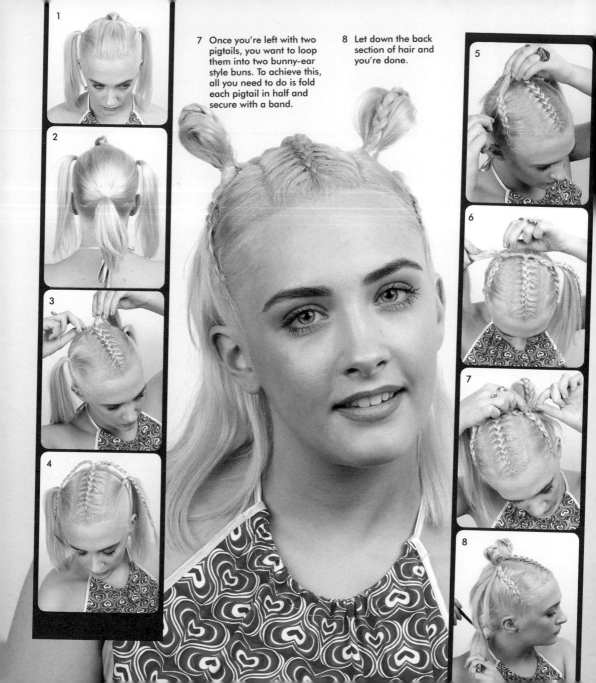

1

2

3

4

7 Once you're left with two pigtails, you want to loop them into two bunny-ear style buns. To achieve this, all you need to do is fold each pigtail in half and secure with a band.

8 Let down the back section of hair and you're done.

5

6

7

8

THE HEADBAND

Step-by-step:

1 Begin with a centre
parting and then create
a front section as shown
in pictures 1 and 1a. Tie
or clip back the remaining
loose hair to keep it out
of the way.

2 Braid one side using the
Dutch Braid technique
(page 16), so that
it frames the face and
tie it off at the ear.

3 Now, repeat step 2
with the opposite side.

Continued overleaf

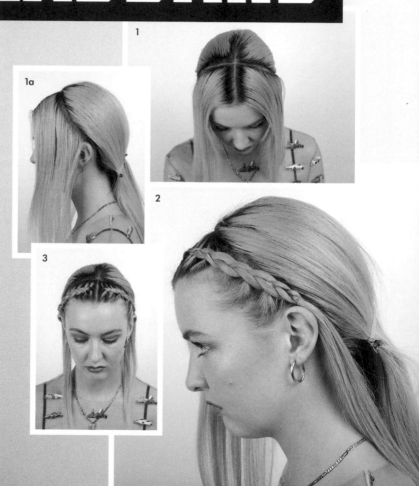

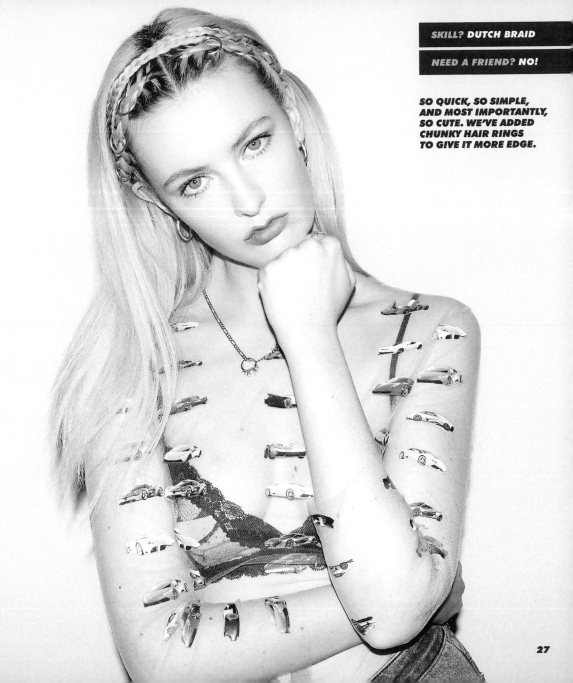

SO QUICK, SO SIMPLE,
AND MOST IMPORTANTLY,
SO CUTE. WE'VE ADDED
CHUNKY HAIR RINGS
TO GIVE IT MORE EDGE.

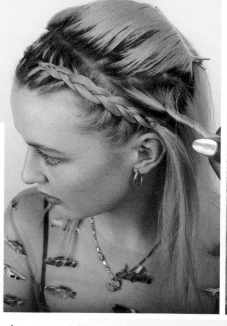

4

4 Unclip the back section of hair and roughly section off a small area of hair behind the ear. Make sure it's thick enough to create a substantial plait. Now, clip or tie back the remaining loose hair again.

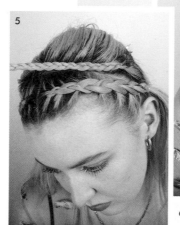

5

5 Plait the new section of hair to the ends and tie off. Cross the plait over to the opposite side of the head (like a headband) and pin down with hair grips behind the ear.

6 Repeat steps 4–5 on the opposite side. Once both plaits are clipped down securely, let down the rest of the hair.

7 If you like, finish with hair rings for extra edge (page 90).

6

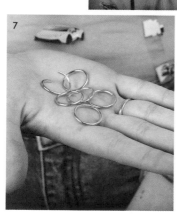

7

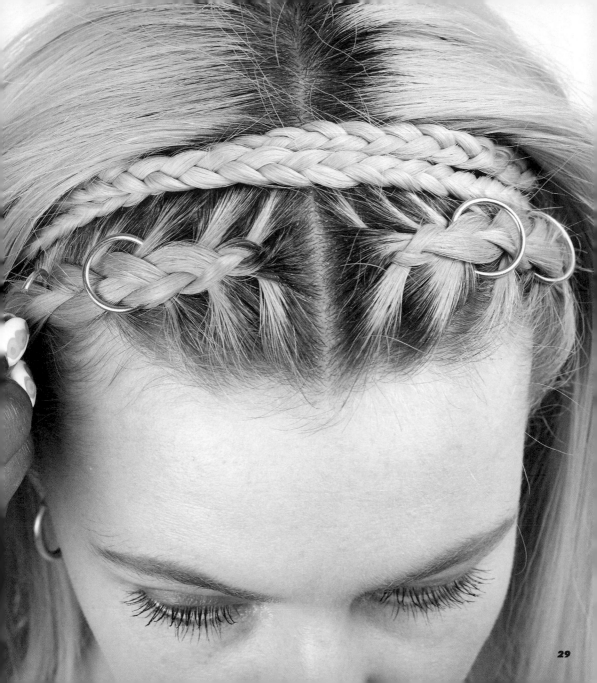

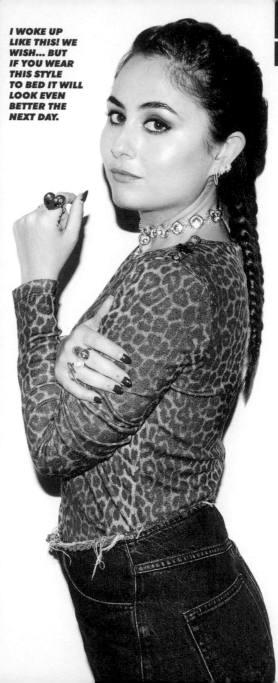
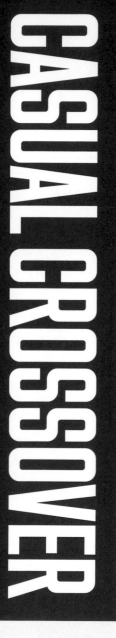

CASUAL CROSSOVER

I WOKE UP LIKE THIS! WE WISH... BUT IF YOU WEAR THIS STYLE TO BED IT WILL LOOK EVEN BETTER THE NEXT DAY.

SKILL? FRENCH BRAID & FISHTAIL PLAIT

NEED A FRIEND? NO!

Step-by-step:

1 Begin with a side parting and continue diagonally to the nape of your neck parting the hair into two sections, as shown in pictures 1 and 1a.

   Note: The parting will finish on the opposite side to where it starts.

2 Begin braiding the smaller section of hair using the French Braid technique (page 14).

3 Continue braiding and tie off at the nape of the neck.

4 Now, begin braiding the other section front-to-back using the French Braid technique (page 14).

5 Tie the braid off at the nape of the neck. It should overlap or rest on top of the first braid.

6 Using the Fishtail Braid technique (page 18), plait the two loose ponytails and tie off.

7 Now, take a pair of scissors and carefully snip and remove the first set of bands used to secure the braids.

8 Using your hands, add some texture to the style by pulling out the braids and plaits to make them more dishevelled. This adds a relaxed and effortless finish to your style.

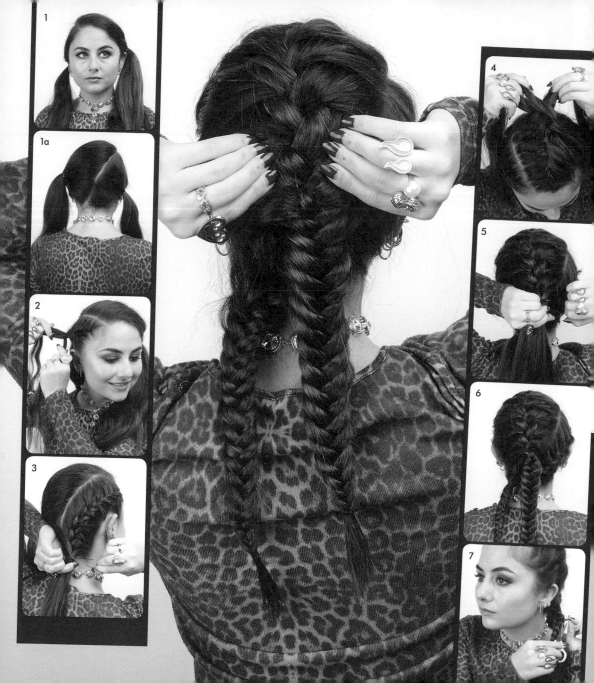

GO FASTER GIRL

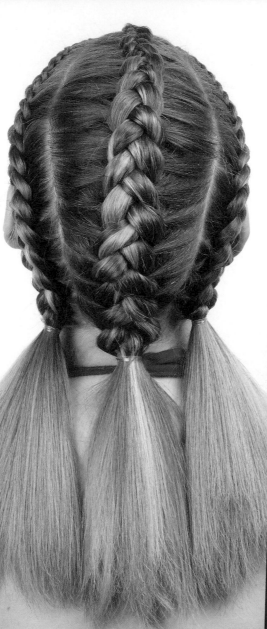

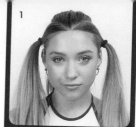

1

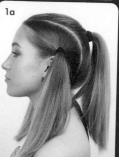

1a

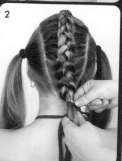

2

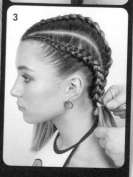

3

Step-by-step:

1 Divide the hair into three sections as shown in pictures 1 and 1a. The middle section of hair should be slightly thicker than the side sections.

Note: The three sections should come to a central point at the hairline as shown in picture 1.

2 Begin braiding the middle section of hair using the Dutch Braid technique (page 16). Aim to keep it as centred as possible and tie the braid off when you reach the nape of the neck.

3 Untie and braid both side sections of hair. Tie them off at the nape of the neck to complete the style.

SKILL? **DUTCH BRAID**

NEED A FRIEND? **YES!**

A FIRM FAVOURITE AT KEASH HQ. CAN'T DECIDE WHETHER YOU WANT TO WEAR YOUR HAIR DOWN OR IN BRAIDS? THIS STYLE TICKS BOTH BOXES.

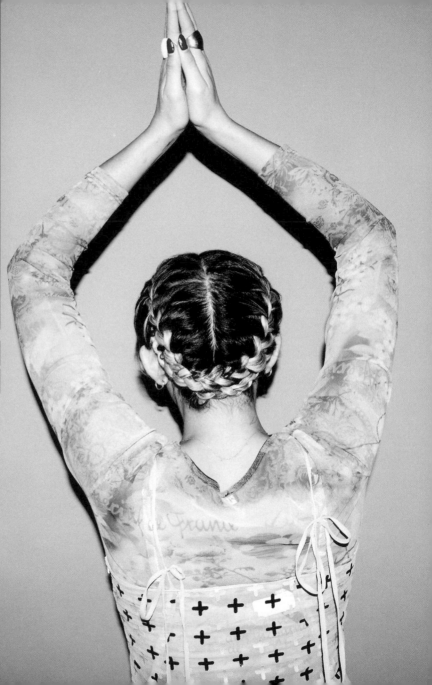

NO ANGEL

THE QUINTESSENTIAL HALO BRAID IS HERE TO STAY, SO HERE IS OUR TAKE ON THE CLASSIC. THIS STYLE WILL STILL LOOK GREAT IN TWO (OR THREE!) DAYS' TIME – IDEAL FOR A FESTIVAL. THE MESSIER THE BETTER, WE SAY!

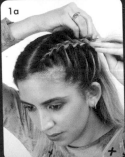

1

1a

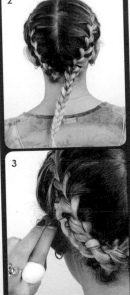

2

3

Step-by-step:

1   Begin by styling your hair into two French braids (page 14).

2   Now, take the left plait and cross it over to the right side and position it next to (slightly tucked under) the right braid. Secure in place using hair grips.

3   Take the right plait and cross it over to the left side and position it next to (slightly tucked under) the left braid. Secure in place using hair grips.

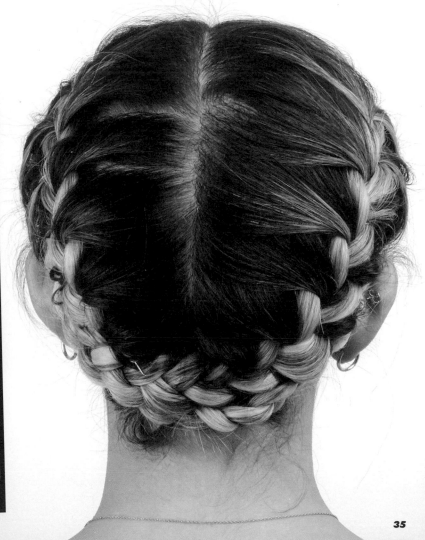

DOUBLE DUTCH

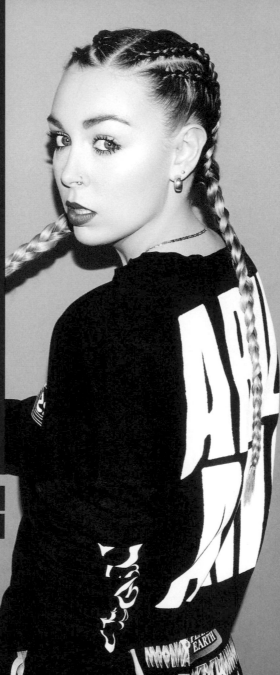

SKILL? DUTCH BRAID

NEED A FRIEND? YES!

ONCE YOU'VE MASTERED DUTCH BRAIDS, THERE'S NO EXCUSE NOT TO GO DOUBLE DUTCH...

Step-by-step:

1 Part the hair into four sections as shown in pictures 1–1b: start with a diagonal side parting and continue down to the nape of the neck with a centre parting, splitting the hair into two sections. Now split these two sections in half to create four sections.

2 Let down one side section of hair, braid using the Dutch Braid technique (page 16) to the nape of the neck and tie off. The braid should be as close as possible to the parting that meets the neighbouring section.

   Tip: Use sectioning clips to keep the neighbouring section of hair out of the way.

3 Now, let down and Dutch Braid (page 16) the neighbouring section of hair to the nape of the neck and tie off. Again, braid the hair as close as possible to the parting that meets the previous section, so both braids are close to each other.

4 Tie the two braids together into one ponytail as shown in picture 4.

5 Repeat steps 2–4 on the remaining sections of hair.

6 Plait both ponytails and tie off at the ends to complete the style. Carefully snip and remove the bands joining the braids into ponytails.

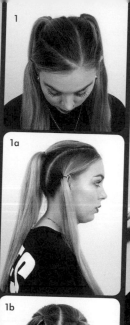

1

1a

1b

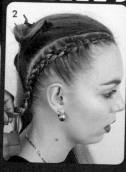

2

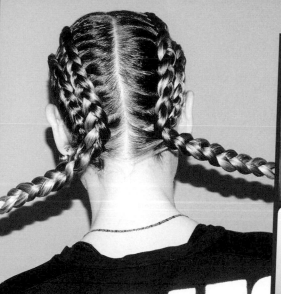

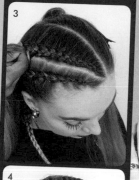

3

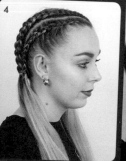

4

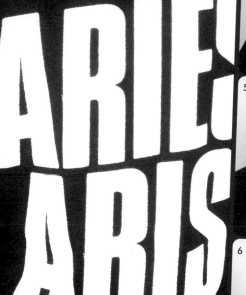

5

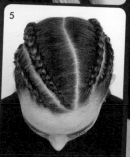

6

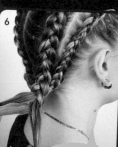

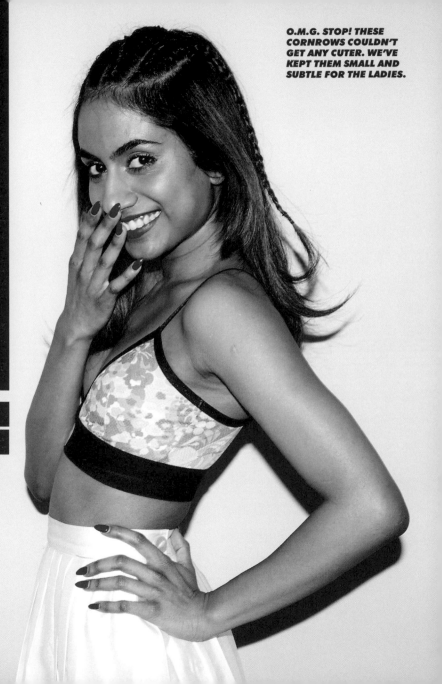

BABY ROWS

SKILL? **FRENCH BRAID**

NEED A FRIEND? **NO!**

O.M.G. STOP! THESE CORNROWS COULDN'T GET ANY CUTER. WE'VE KEPT THEM SMALL AND SUBTLE FOR THE LADIES.

Step-by-step:

1 Part the front section of hair into four equally sized sections as shown in picture 1.

2 Untie one section and begin braiding front-to-back using the French Braid technique (page 14). Start with the side sections and work your way to the middle section.

3 Once the braid reaches the end of the section, continue plaiting the hair and tie it off at the end.

4 Repeat steps 2–3 with the remaining three sections.

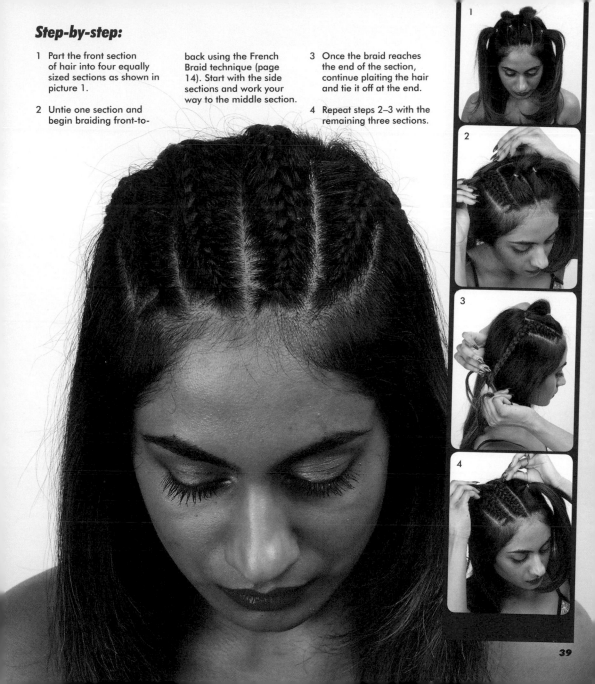

39

WAVY BRAIDS

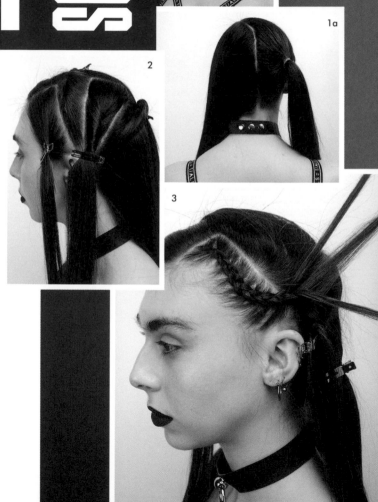

1

1a

2

3

Step-by-step:

1 Create a diagonal side
   parting and continue to
   the nape of the neck,
   ending with a centre
   parting as shown in
   pictures 1 and 1a. Tie off
   one half of the hair to
   keep it out of the way.

2 Part the loose side of hair
   into five sections and clip
   the sections in alternating
   directions.

   Note: The hair is clipped
   in the direction of the
   braid, with the section
   closest to the face clipped
   downwards.

3 Unclip the front section
   of hair (closest to the face)
   and begin braiding from
   top-to-bottom, using the
   Dutch Braid technique
   (page 16). When you
   reach the bottom of the
   first section, unclip the
   neighbouring section and
   curve the braid 'around
   the corner' to join the
   new section of hair.

   Continued overleaf

40

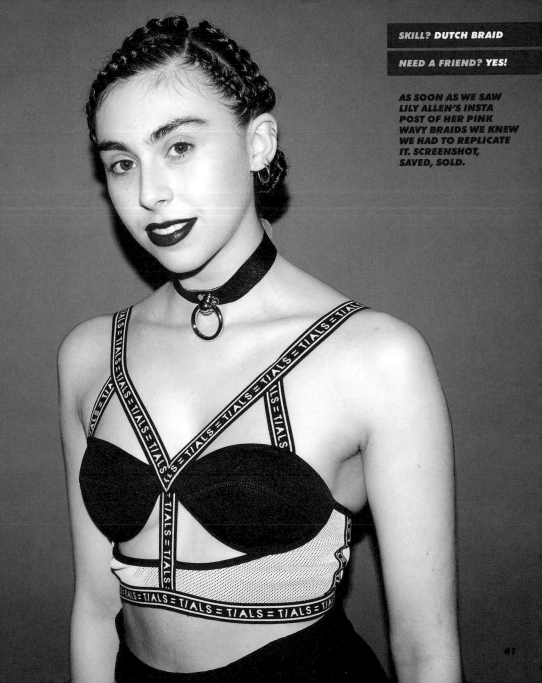

AS SOON AS WE SAW
LILY ALLEN'S INSTA
POST OF HER PINK
WAVY BRAIDS WE KNEW
WE HAD TO REPLICATE
IT. SCREENSHOT,
SAVED, SOLD.

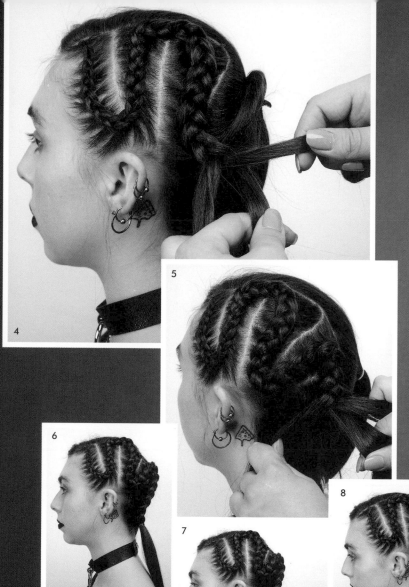

4 Continue braiding in this motion – unclipping the neighbouring section as you reach the end of the current section.

5 Once you reach the final section of hair at the back of the head make sure to pick up and include all loose hair in the braid.

6 Once the final section is braided, tie it off at the nape of your neck.

7 Plait the loose ponytail and tie it off.

8 Create a bun at the nape of your neck by twisting and wrapping the loose plait around.

9 Fasten your bun with hair grips and bands. Make sure it feels secure!

Repeat steps 2–9 with the other half of your hair.

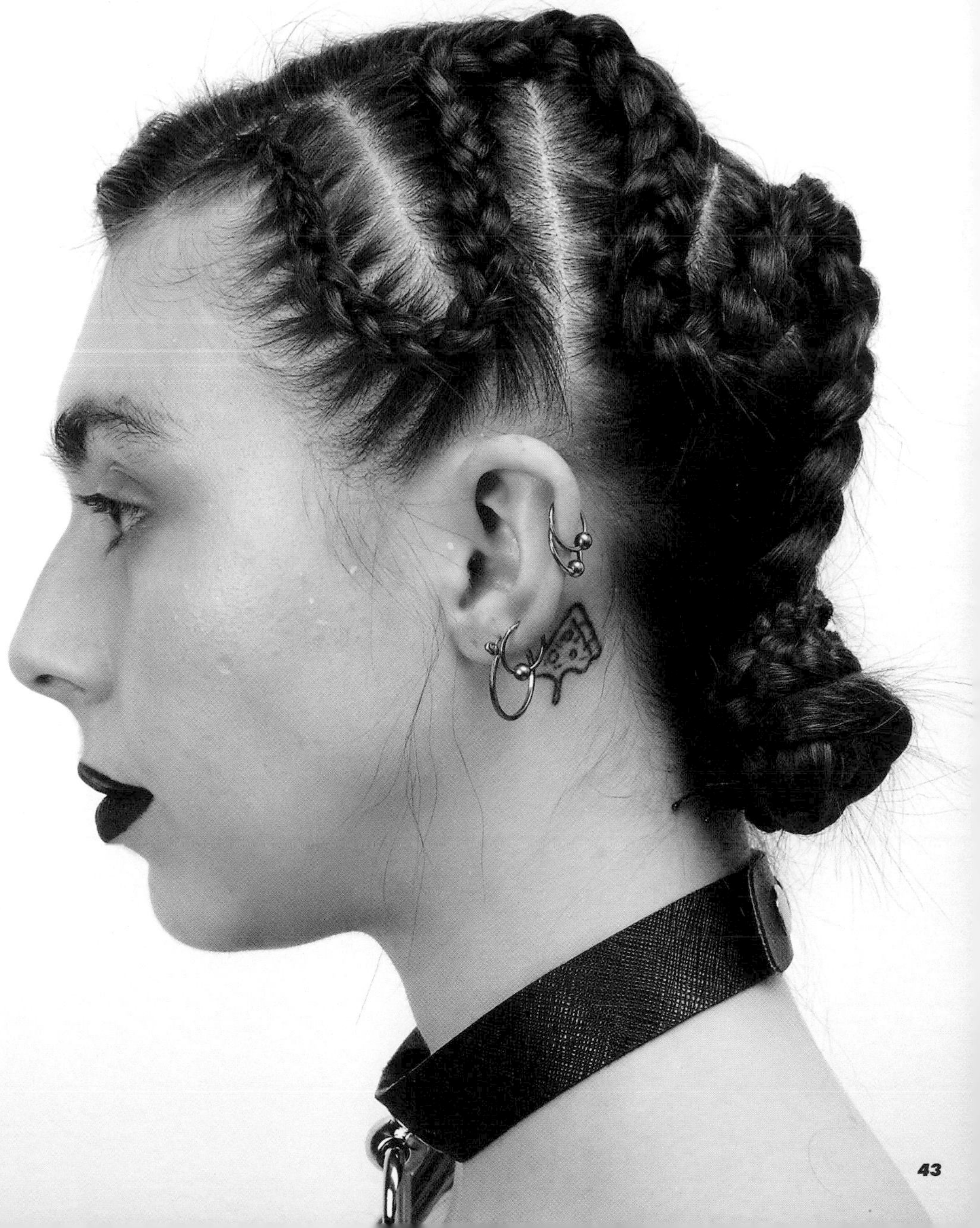

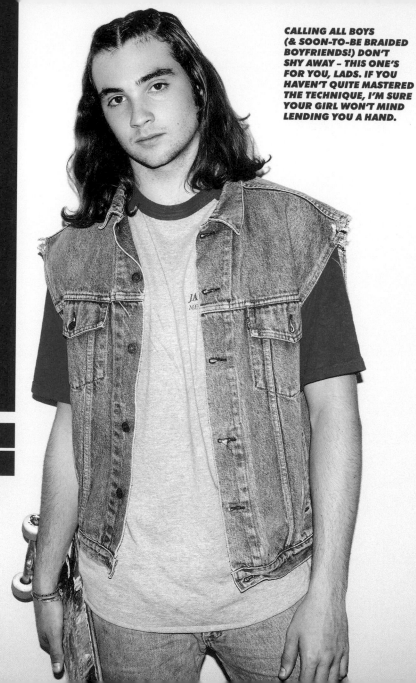

BOY BRAIDS

PT. 1

SKILL? **FRENCH BRAID**

NEED A FRIEND? **NO!**

CALLING ALL BOYS (& SOON-TO-BE BRAIDED BOYFRIENDS!) DON'T SHY AWAY – THIS ONE'S FOR YOU, LADS. IF YOU HAVEN'T QUITE MASTERED THE TECHNIQUE, I'M SURE YOUR GIRL WON'T MIND LENDING YOU A HAND.

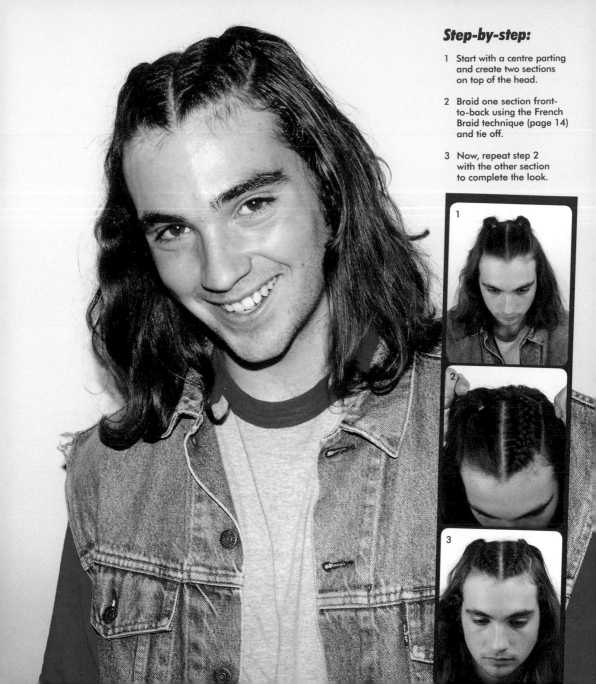

Step-by-step:

1 Start with a centre parting and create two sections on top of the head.

2 Braid one section front-to-back using the French Braid technique (page 14) and tie off.

3 Now, repeat step 2 with the other section to complete the look.

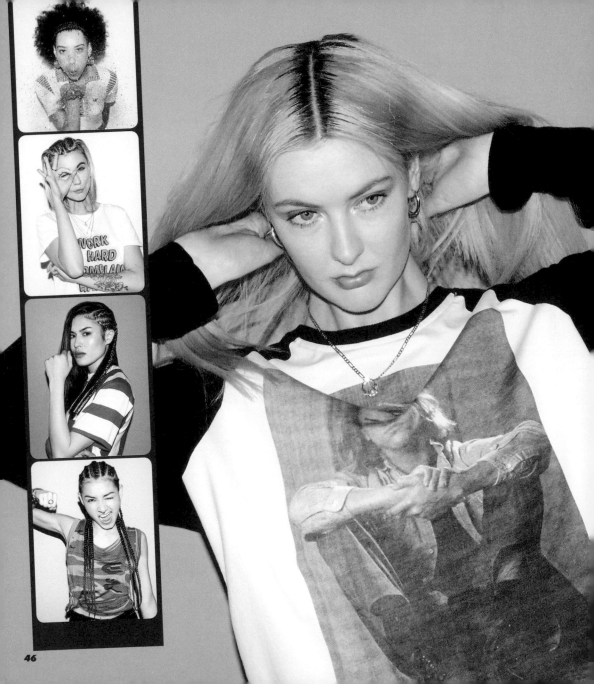

WANT TO BRIGHTEN UP YOUR BRAIDS? THIS SECTION DEMONSTRATES HOW YOU CAN EXPERIMENT WITH QUICK, EASY AND FUN WAYS TO ADD COLOUR TO YOUR BRAIDS.

Colouring Kit:

Our Colouring Kit is ideal for those who like to change up their hair in no time. Add some extra personality with coloured hair strips, brighten up your braids with hair chalk or add sparkle with a sprinkle of glitter.

Coloured hair chalks are a great temporary hair colour solution that are readily available in a whole heap of shades. We use sticks and domes to create our desired effect. Domes are a great no-mess option – you can apply it directly onto the hair without getting it all over your hands. Hair chalk sticks are great when you're feeling experimental – check out our DIY Hair Paint tutorial (page 52).

For more precise application of colour we recommend hair pens, as you can take a lot more care when applying the colour. They're great for colouring in braids as you can be accurate in your application for a cleaner finish.

Now, last but not least, up the ante with glitter. Whether you want to apply it to your braids or your roots, we recommend getting yourself both chunky and fine glitter in a variety of colours. See our Glitter tutorial on page 50.

1 Fudge Urban Hair Chalk Domes
  (Electrik Blue, Pumped Up Purple & Festival Pink)
2 Ombre Hair Chalk Set from Urban Outfitters
3 Pixie Lott Paint Hair Chalk Pens (Pink & Blue)
4 In Your Dreams Chunky Glitter
5 Loose Fine Glitter

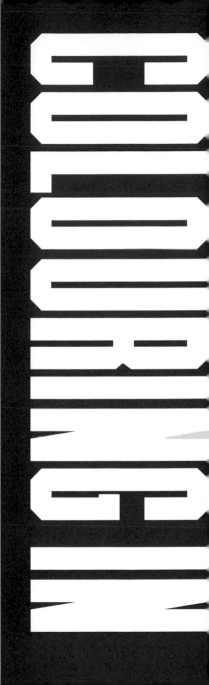

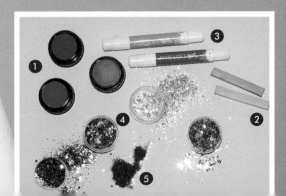

CHALK & CRAYONS

Step-by-step:

1 You can use hair chalk or hair chalk pens to colour your style. We like to use hair chalk pens to colour the braid as you can be more precise when applying the colour.

   Tip: Use different shades to create a faded or ombre effect.

2 If you fancy adding colour to the rest of the hair, we suggest using hair chalk domes or sticks. Their dry consistency works well on loose hair and is really easy to apply.

3 We like to add random streaks of colour throughout and create a dip-dye effect by chalking the ends of the hair.

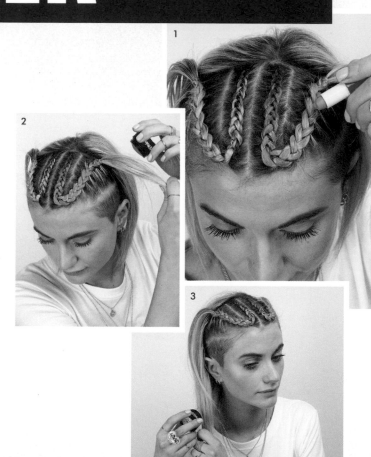

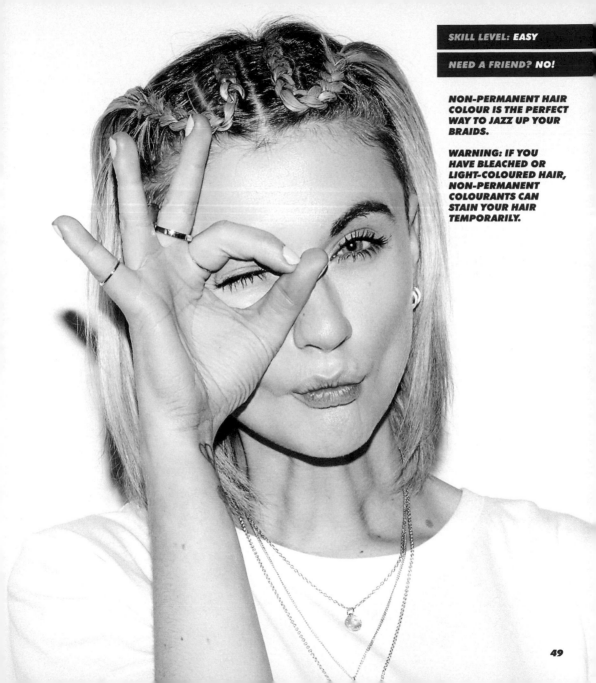

NON-PERMANENT HAIR COLOUR IS THE PERFECT WAY TO JAZZ UP YOUR BRAIDS.

WARNING: IF YOU HAVE BLEACHED OR LIGHT-COLOURED HAIR, NON-PERMANENT COLOURANTS CAN STAIN YOUR HAIR TEMPORARILY.

49

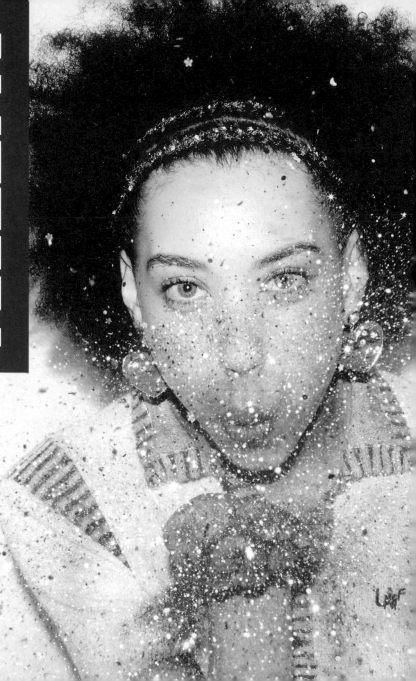

GLITTER!

ADDING GLITTER TO
YOUR BRAIDS IS QUICK
AND EASY! WE LIKE TO
MIX IT UP AND USE FINE
AND CHUNKY GLITTER...

Step-by-step:

1 Squeeze a small amount of hair gel into your hand.

2 Use your fingertips to apply the hair gel onto the braids where you want to add the glitter.

Tip: Put a towel around your shoulders so you don't get glitter on your top.

3 Pour some loose glitter onto a surface or empty lid.

4 Again using your fingertips, apply glitter to the gelled braids. Spray a layer of hairspray over the glitter to hold it in place.

Tip: Make a glitter and gel mix to create your own DIY glitter paste. Just add a squeeze of hair gel and as much or as little glitter as you want and mix together with your fingers.

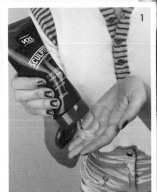

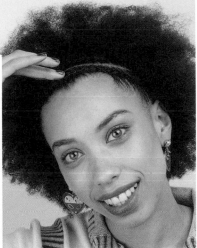

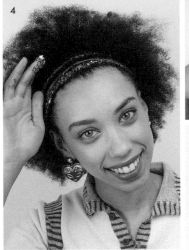

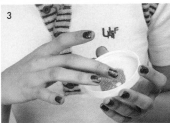

SKILL LEVEL: EASY

NEED A FRIEND? NO!

TIP: MAKE SURE TO HAVE SOME MAKE-UP WIPES OR TISSUES CLOSE BY BECAUSE THIS CAN GET MESSY!

RAINBOW ROOTS

Step-by-step:

1 Use the mortar and pestle to crush the chalk into a fine dust. Using a paintbrush, mix in a small amount of hair gel and water to create a paste-like consistency.

   Note: Too much water and gel will make the colour less intense.

2 Once you've created your coloured paint paste, apply to a small section at the roots, using a paintbrush.

   Tip: Use a mirror to see what you're doing!

3 Apply the paint colour by colour, making sure to rinse your brush thoroughly between each colour change. Alternate the colours to create a rainbow effect.

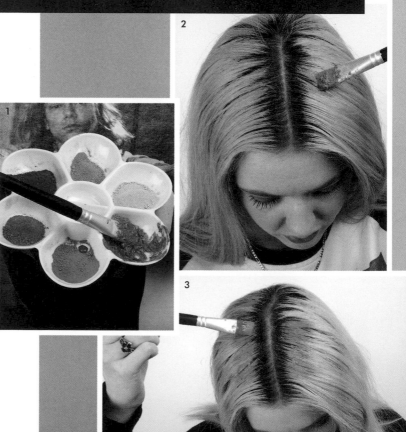

TAKE YOUR ART SKILLS TO THE NEXT LEVEL AND PREPARE TO GET YOUR HANDS DIRTY WITH OUR DIY HAIR PAINT. DIG OUT YOUR PAINTBRUSHES – IT'S A RECIPE FOR SUCCESS!

SKILL LEVEL: EASY

NEED A FRIEND? NO!

Rainbow Roots Kit:

Raid your bedroom and your mum's kitchen for these household essentials. We use a mortar and pestle to crush up hair chalk sticks quickly and easily. You'll also need a plate or paint palette to mix up your paints, a wide, flat paintbrush and a pot of water to rinse your brush.

1 Hair Chalk Sticks
2 Hair Gel
3 Mortar & Pestle
4 Paint Palette
5 Paintbrush (roughly 2 cm/¾ in)
6 Pot of water

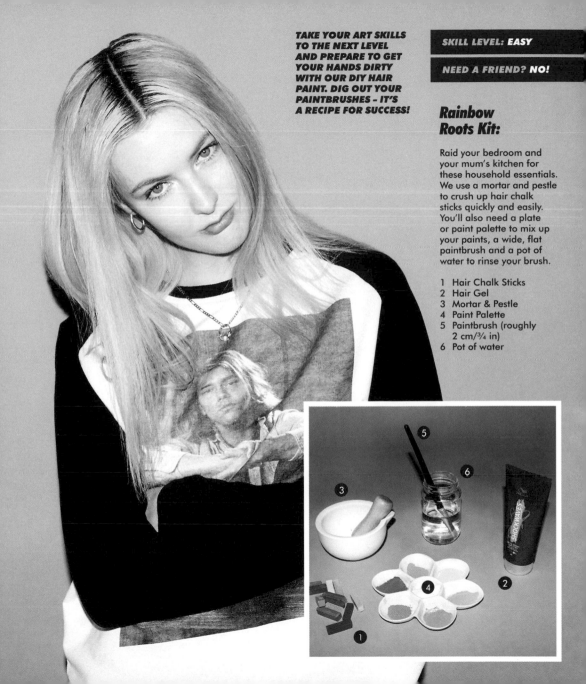

OMBRE BRAIDS

DIP DYE YOUR BRAIDS IN FOUR QUICK AND EASY STEPS. DECIDING WHICH COLOUR WILL BE THE HARDEST PART...

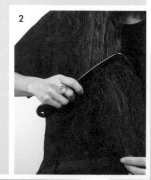

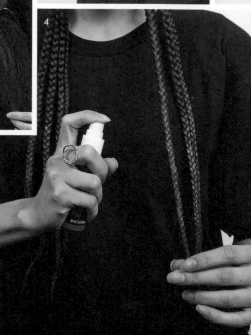

Step-by-step:

1 To begin, throw on an old T-shirt or wrap a towel around your shoulders as this can get quite messy. Split your hair in half and apply coloured hairspray (or hair chalk) to the ends of the hair to create a dip-dyed effect.

   Note: If you have light-coloured hair, you don't need to apply colour before braiding. You can skip ahead to step 4.

2 Once you've got decent colour coverage, brush through the hair with a wide tooth comb to eliminate knots.

   Note: This will brush out some colour.

3 Repeat steps 1–2 for the remaining half of hair.

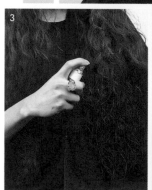

4 Now braid the hair – we've gone for Boy Braids Pt. 2 (page 86), then re-apply coloured hairspray (or hair chalk) to the ends for maximum impact.

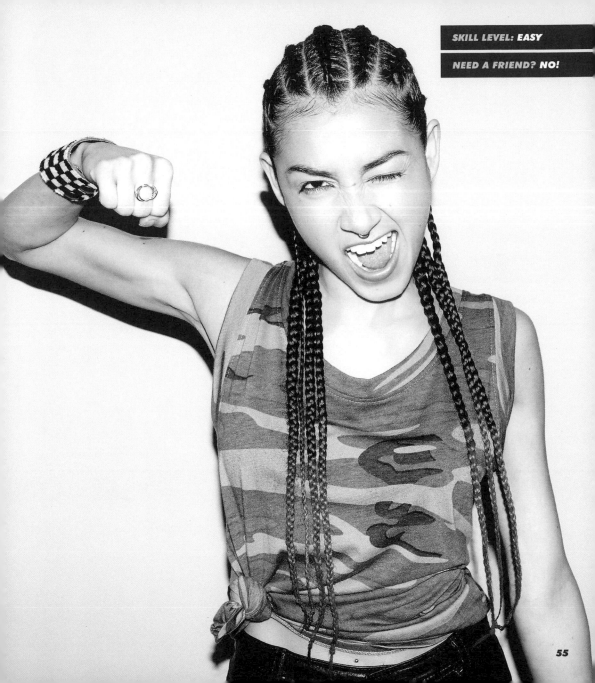

KILLER CORNROWS

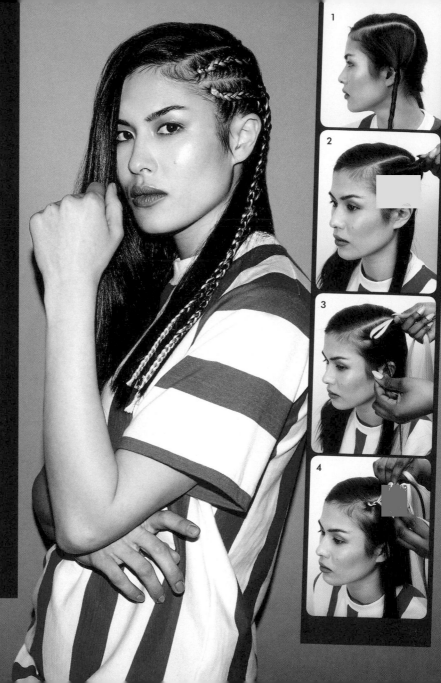

Step-by-step:

1 Begin with a side parting then neatly section off a small area of hair as shown in picture 1. Tie the remaining loose hair to one side to keep it out of the way.

2 Split the section in half, making sure both sections are of equal width, and clip the lower section down to keep it out of the way.

3 Now add in the coloured hair strip. The strip should be roughly 1 cm (½ in) thick. Take a small strand of hair from the hairline and loop the hair strip around the strand as shown in picture 3. Tightly tie the coloured hair strip in a tight knot around the strand of hair to secure it.

Tip: If you're struggling, try using a thinner strip of coloured hair.

4 You will have three strands of hair to work with. Two strands will be the coloured hair strip and the third strand will be your own hair. Begin to braid using the Dutch Braid technique (page 16), picking up hair from the scalp as you go.

Tip: Pinch and pull the strands tight to create a neater finish.

5 Continue braiding to the end of the section. Once you can't braid any further, you can either tie off at this point or continue with a loose plait to the ends of the hair, as we have.

6 Unclip the lower section of hair and repeat steps 3–5.

A BRAIDED UNDERCUT IS A CLASSIC. NOW ADD MORE EDGE TO YOUR UNDERCUT WITH COLOURED HAIR STRIPS. YOU CAN FIND A LARGE RANGE OF COLOURED SYNTHETIC HAIR EXTENSIONS AT COSMETIC SHOPS. IT'S BEST TO BUY LOOSE WEAVE (NOT ON TRACKS). ONCE YOU'VE GOT THE HANG OF IT YOU'LL BE ADDING HAIR STRIPS TO ALL YOUR BRAIDS. TRUST US, WE'VE BEEN THERE.

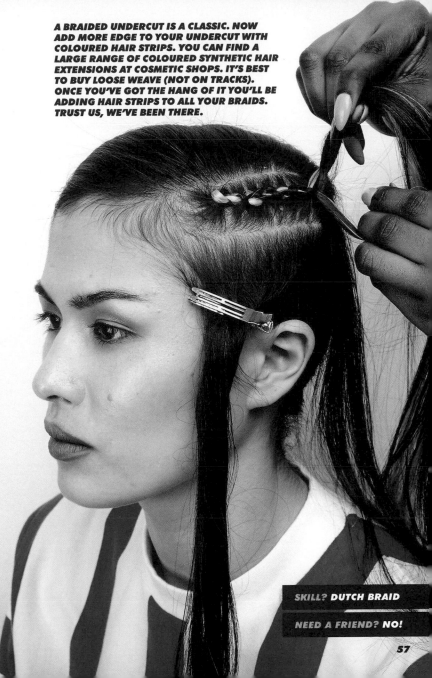

SKILL? **DUTCH BRAID**

NEED A FRIEND? **NO!**

WHO IS YOUR KEASH BRAIDS! QUEEN?

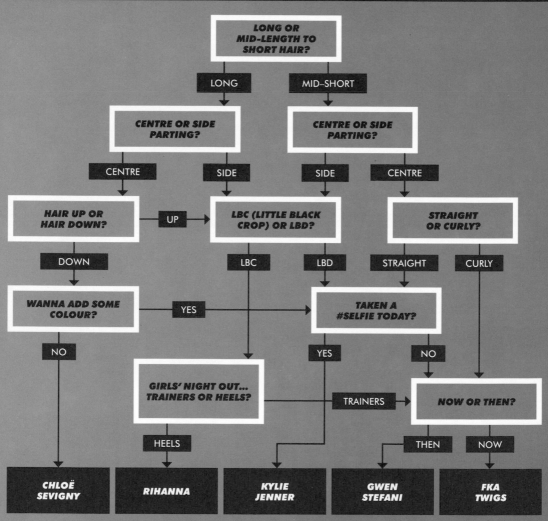

LONG OR MID-LENGTH TO SHORT HAIR?

LONG → **CENTRE OR SIDE PARTING?**

MID–SHORT → **CENTRE OR SIDE PARTING?**

CENTRE → **HAIR UP OR HAIR DOWN?**

SIDE → **LBC (LITTLE BLACK CROP) OR LBD?**

SIDE → **LBC (LITTLE BLACK CROP) OR LBD?**

CENTRE → **STRAIGHT OR CURLY?**

UP → LBC/LBD

DOWN → **WANNA ADD SOME COLOUR?**

LBC → **GIRLS' NIGHT OUT... TRAINERS OR HEELS?**

LBD → **TAKEN A #SELFIE TODAY?**

STRAIGHT → **TAKEN A #SELFIE TODAY?**

CURLY → **NOW OR THEN?**

YES → **TAKEN A #SELFIE TODAY?**

NO → **CHLOË SEVIGNY**

YES → **GIRLS' NIGHT OUT... TRAINERS OR HEELS?**

TRAINERS → **NOW OR THEN?**

HEELS → **RIHANNA**

YES → **KYLIE JENNER**

NO → **NOW OR THEN?**

THEN → **GWEN STEFANI**

NOW → **FKA TWIGS**

58

FIND OUT WHICH HAIRSTYLES ARE RIGHT FOR YOU WITH OUR QUICK AND EASY QUIZ. READY, SET, GO!

CHLOË SEVIGNY

Strike that cute but cool balance, recreating classic styles with a twist. Keep it carefree and nonchalant.

Suggested styles:
The Headband (page 26)
No Angel (page 34)
The Heart (page 100)
Dutch Braids (page 16)

RIHANNA

A bad gal style chameleon, you need a new look for every day of the week and we totally get it.

Suggested styles:
Bad Gal Buns (page 106)
Hella High Pony (page 70)
Wavy Pony (page 82)
Rope Braid (page 20)

KYLIE JENNER

Pout those lips, do your squats, braid your hair and most importantly apply your lippy. Time for a #selfie!

Suggested styles:
Killer Cornrows (page 56)
Go Faster Girl (page 32)
Casual Crossover (page 30)
Boy Braids Pt. 2 (page 86)

GWEN STEFANI

Got a penchant for '90s nostalgia? Cornrows, space buns and hair chalk are your new style go-tos.

Suggested styles:
Baby Rows (page 38)
Baby Girl Buns (page 62)
Chalk & Crayons (page 48)
Playgirl Bunny (page 24)

FKA TWIGS

You'd rather go avant-garde than au natural. All hail Braid Queen Twigs – the mother of all hair envy.

Suggested styles:
TWIGS (page 72)
Wavy Braids (page 40)
Kiss Curls (page 96)
The Star (page 104)

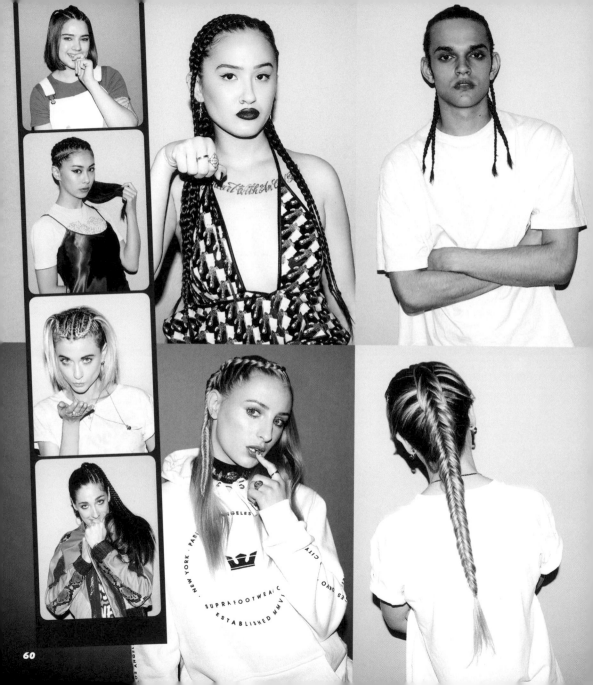

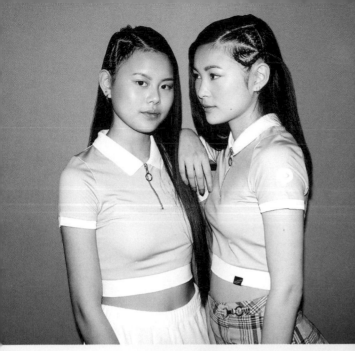

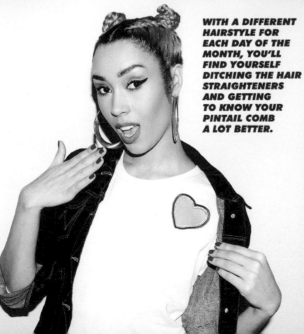

WITH A DIFFERENT HAIRSTYLE FOR EACH DAY OF THE MONTH, YOU'LL FIND YOURSELF DITCHING THE HAIR STRAIGHTENERS AND GETTING TO KNOW YOUR PINTAIL COMB A LOT BETTER.

THE BRAIDS

PART 2

BABY GIRL BUNS

Step-by-step:

1 Start with a centre parting and continue this to the nape of your neck, splitting your hair in half. Now split both sides in half to create four equally sized sections as shown in pictures 1–1b.

2 Let down one of the front sections and braid front-to-back using the Dutch Braid technique (page 16). Continue with a plait to the ends of the hair and then tie off.

Continued overleaf

1

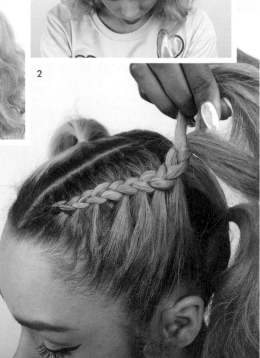

1a

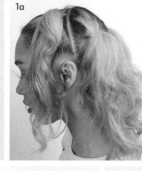

2

1b

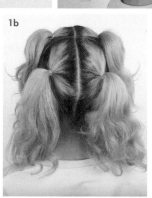

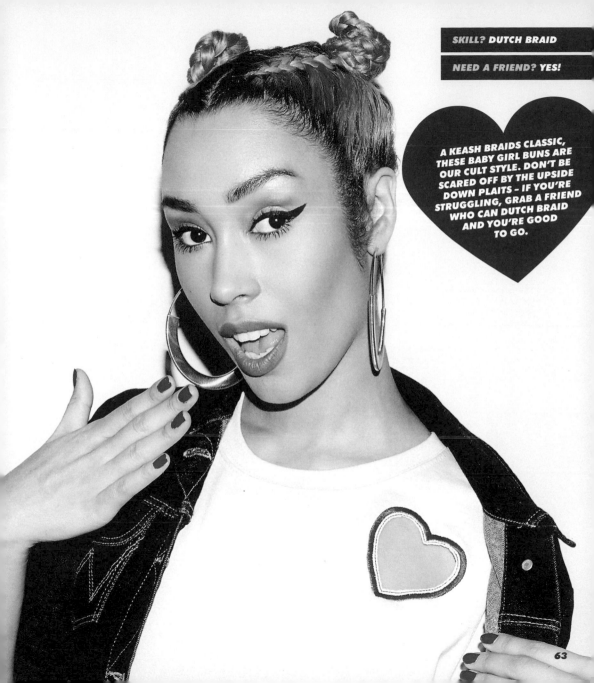

A KEASH BRAIDS CLASSIC, THESE BABY GIRL BUNS ARE OUR CULT STYLE. DON'T BE SCARED OFF BY THE UPSIDE DOWN PLAITS - IF YOU'RE STRUGGLING, GRAB A FRIEND WHO CAN DUTCH BRAID AND YOU'RE GOOD TO GO.

63

3 Repeat step 2 with the other front section.

4 Now, it's time to braid the back sections using the same Dutch Braid technique (page 16). It can be slightly awkward, but it's worth it! Repeat step 2 for both sections but braiding from the neck upwards.

Tip: If you're braiding your friends hair get them to rest their head face-down on their lap.

5 Tie the two left plaits together, and then tie the two right plaits together, to create two plaited ponytails.

6 Twist the left ponytail into a bun and secure with hair grips and bands as neatly as you can.

7 Repeat step 6 with the right ponytail.

3

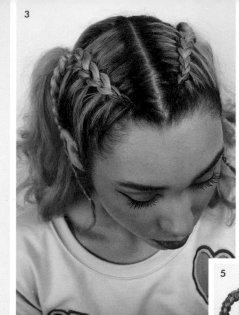

4

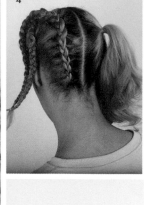

5

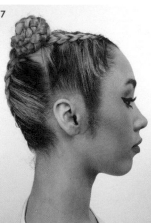

6

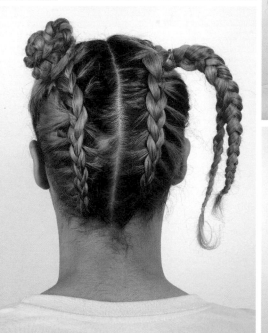

7

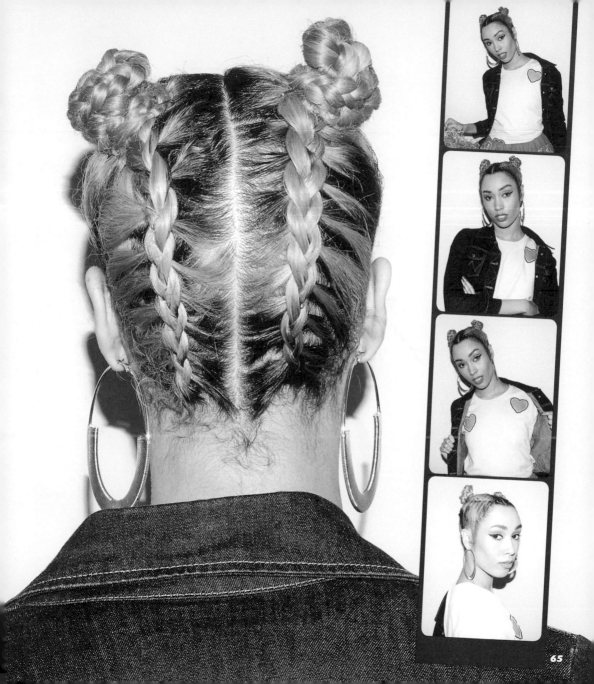

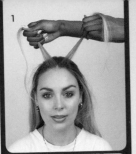

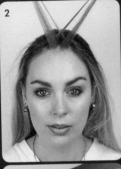

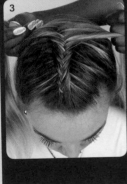

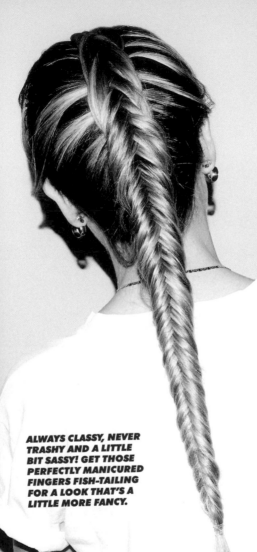

ALWAYS CLASSY, NEVER TRASHY AND A LITTLE BIT SASSY! GET THOSE PERFECTLY MANICURED FINGERS FISH-TAILING FOR A LOOK THAT'S A LITTLE MORE FANCY.

Step-by-step:

1 Pick up a section of hair from the middle of the forehead, roughly 3 cm (1¼ in) wide. Split this section in half – like the Fishtail Plait (page 18), this technique only requires two strands.

2 Separate a small strand of hair from the outer edge of the left strand, cross it under and add it to the right strand. Re-grip and pull apart both strands to tighten the plait – you should still be holding two strands.

Now, separate a small strand of hair from the outer edge of the right strand, cross it under and add it to the left strand. Again, re-grip and pull apart both strands to tighten the plait.

3 Take a small strand of hair from the outer edge of the left strand and pick up a small section of loose hair from the left side. Cross these under and add to the right strand. Pull the strands apart to keep the plait tight.

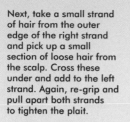

Next, take a small strand of hair from the outer edge of the right strand and pick up a small section of loose hair from the scalp. Cross these under and add to the left strand. Again, re-grip and pull apart both strands to tighten the plait.

4 Repeat step 3 until you reach the nape of the neck. From the nape of the neck, continue with a Fishtail Plait (page 18) until you reach the ends of the hair. Tie off to complete the look.

Tip: If you find this style difficult, practice on a smaller section of hair to master the technique.

FISHTAIL DUTCH

SKILL? *FISHTAIL DUTCH & FISHTAIL PLAIT*

NEED A FRIEND? YES!

Step-by-step:

1 Begin with a side parting. Then, create a half-circle parting as shown in picture 1, and tie off the remaining loose hair to keep it out of the way.

2 Split the section into two sections with a diagonal parting.

3 Clip the top section out of the way and split the lower section into two halves with a diagonal parting.

4 Begin by braiding the front section back-to-front using the Dutch Braid technique (page 16).

5 When the braid reaches the hairline, unclip the neighbouring section and curve the braid 'around the corner' to join the next section of hair. Continue braiding the new section along your hairline, framing your face.

6 When the braid reaches the ear, begin to angle it upwards to create a half heart shape. When you have completed braiding the section, tie it off.

7 Now, create the same half heart shape with the top section of hair. Begin by unclipping the top section and splitting it into two sections.

8 Repeat step 4. When the braid reaches the hairline, unclip the neighbouring section and curve the braid 'around the corner' to join the new section of hair.

SKILL? **DUTCH BRAID**

NEED A FRIEND? **YES!**

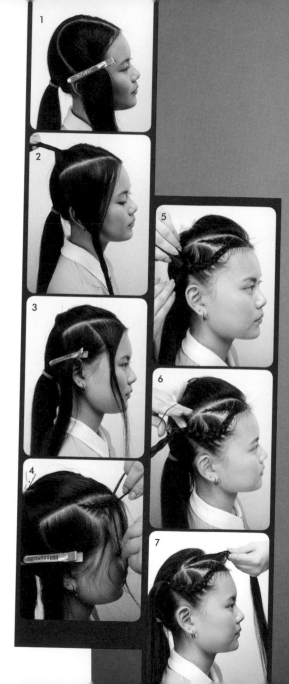

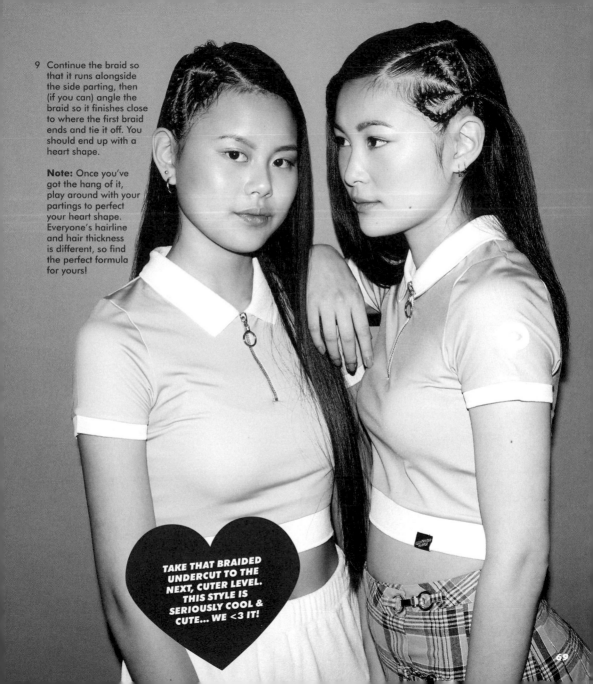

9 Continue the braid so that it runs alongside the side parting, then (if you can) angle the braid so it finishes close to where the first braid ends and tie it off. You should end up with a heart shape.

Note: Once you've got the hang of it, play around with your partings to perfect your heart shape. Everyone's hairline and hair thickness is different, so find the perfect formula for yours!

TAKE THAT BRAIDED UNDERCUT TO THE NEXT, CUTER LEVEL. THIS STYLE IS SERIOUSLY COOL & CUTE... WE <3 IT!

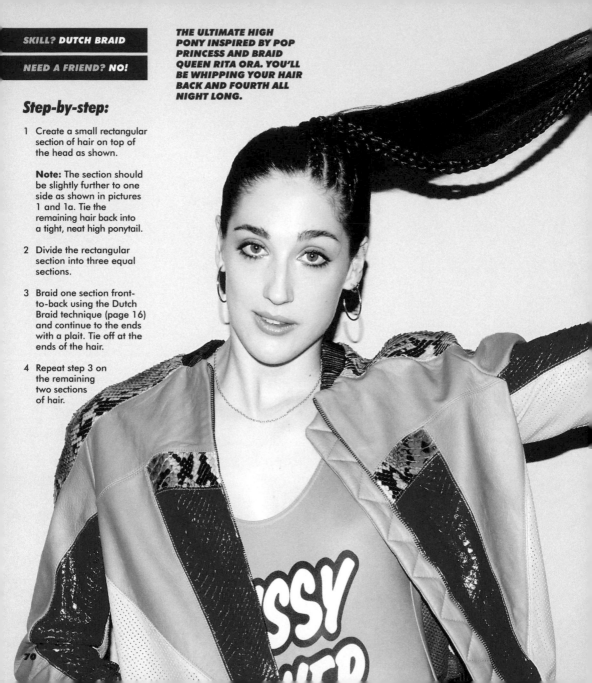

THE ULTIMATE HIGH PONY INSPIRED BY POP PRINCESS AND BRAID QUEEN RITA ORA. YOU'LL BE WHIPPING YOUR HAIR BACK AND FOURTH ALL NIGHT LONG.

Step-by-step:

1 Create a small rectangular section of hair on top of the head as shown.

   Note: The section should be slightly further to one side as shown in pictures 1 and 1a. Tie the remaining hair back into a tight, neat high ponytail.

2 Divide the rectangular section into three equal sections.

3 Braid one section front-to-back using the Dutch Braid technique (page 16) and continue to the ends with a plait. Tie off at the ends of the hair.

4 Repeat step 3 on the remaining two sections of hair.

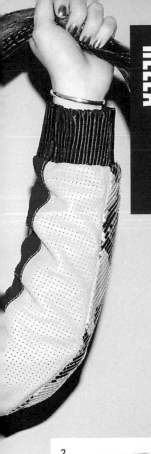

HELLA HIGH PONY

1
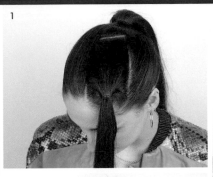

1a
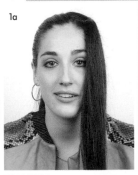

2
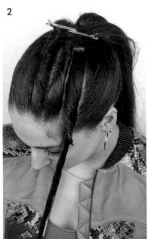

3
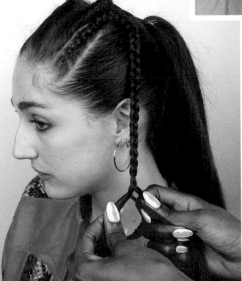

4
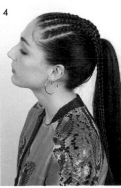

TWIGS

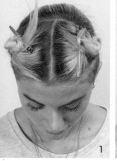

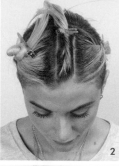

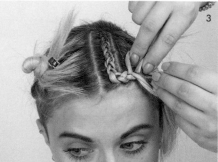

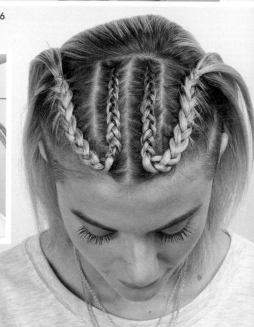

Step-by-step:

1 Begin with a centre parting. Now, create two sections on top of the head as shown in picture 1. Both section should finish 2–3 cm (¾–1¾ in) above the ears. Tie back the remaining loose hair to keep out of the way.

2 Unclip one section and create a new parting as shown in picture 2.

Note: The new section should be roughly a third of the whole section.

3 Begin braiding the new section back-to-front, using the Dutch Braid technique (page 16). When you reach the hairline you need to curve the braid 'around the corner' to join the neighbouring section of hair and reposition your hands to braid in the opposite direction.

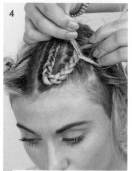

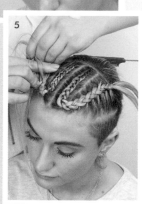

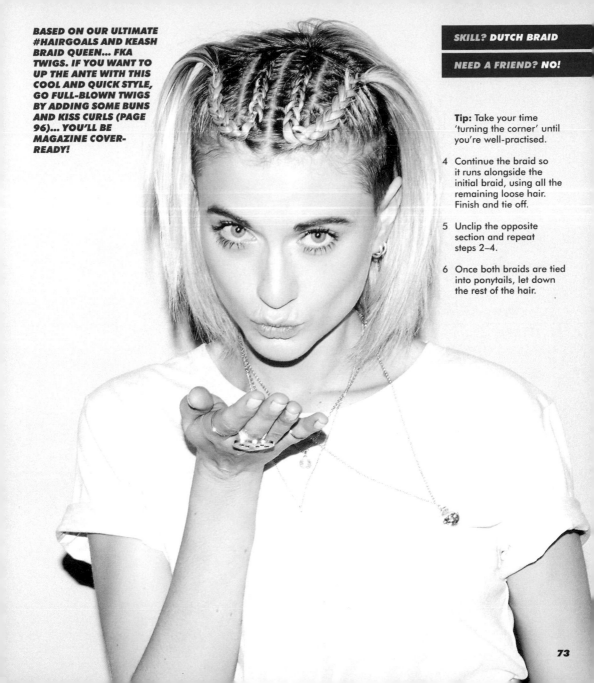

BASED ON OUR ULTIMATE #HAIRGOALS AND KEASH BRAID QUEEN... FKA TWIGS. IF YOU WANT TO UP THE ANTE WITH THIS COOL AND QUICK STYLE, GO FULL-BLOWN TWIGS BY ADDING SOME BUNS AND KISS CURLS (PAGE 96)... YOU'LL BE MAGAZINE COVER-READY!

SKILL? DUTCH BRAID

NEED A FRIEND? NO!

Tip: Take your time 'turning the corner' until you're well-practised.

4 Continue the braid so it runs alongside the initial braid, using all the remaining loose hair. Finish and tie off.

5 Unclip the opposite section and repeat steps 2–4.

6 Once both braids are tied into ponytails, let down the rest of the hair.

TRIPLE TROUBLE

1 Part the top section of hair into three sections as shown in pictures 1 and 1a.

   Note: The middle section should be thicker than the two side sections and the partings should be slightly curved. Tie or clip back the remaining loose hair to keep out of the way.

2 Braid the middle section of hair front-to-back using the Dutch Braid technique (page 16) and tie off into a ponytail.

   Note: Aim to keep your braid as centred as you can.

3 Now, braid both side sections and tie off, to complete the look.

SKILL? DUTCH BRAID

NEED A FRIEND? NO!

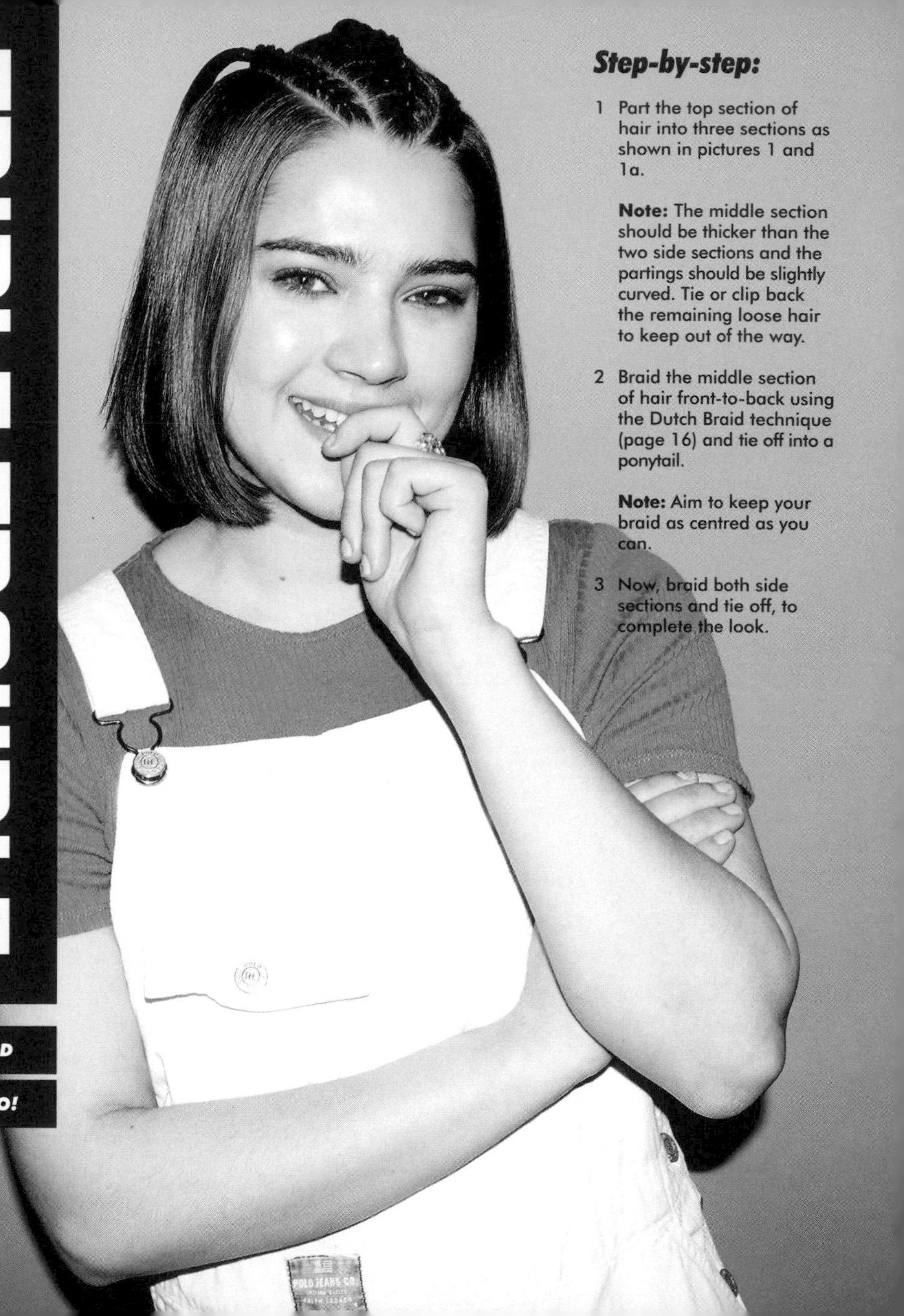

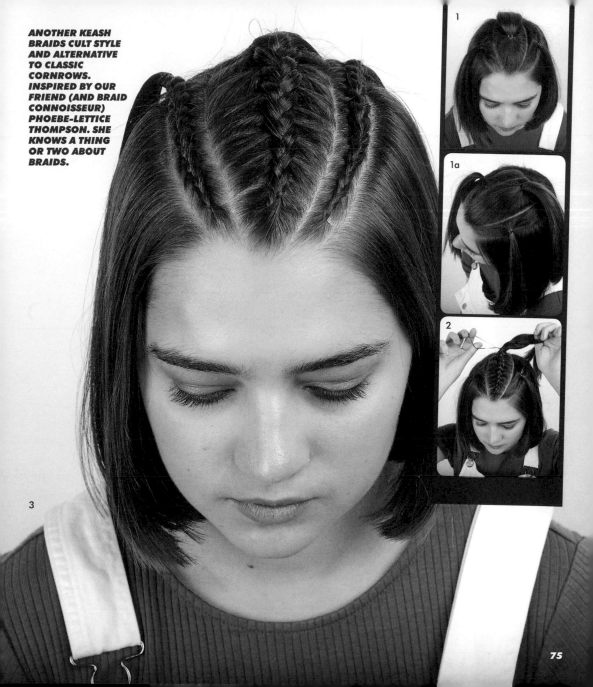

ANOTHER KEASH
BRAIDS CULT STYLE
AND ALTERNATIVE
TO CLASSIC
CORNROWS.
INSPIRED BY OUR
FRIEND (AND BRAID
CONNOISSEUR)
PHOEBE-LETTICE
THOMPSON. SHE
KNOWS A THING
OR TWO ABOUT
BRAIDS.

1

1a

2

3

ON POINT

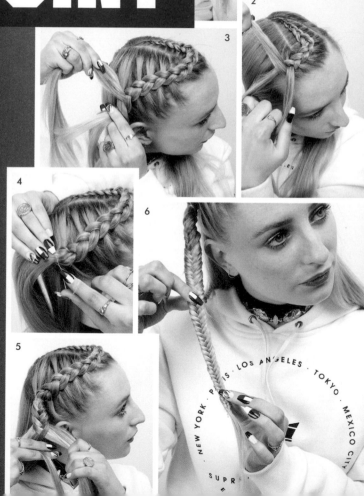

Step-by-step:

1   Begin by creating a triangular section of hair on top of the head as shown in picture 1.

    Tip: Clip down the loose hair on both sides to keep it out of the way.

2   Using the Dutch Braid technique (page 16), begin braiding back-to-front, starting at the top of the head.

3   When the braid reaches the hairline, unclip the right side of loose hair and curve the braid 'around the corner' to join the right section of hair.

    Note: You can unclip and braid the left side if you'd prefer!

4   Continue braiding the new section of hair, angling the braid downwards. Tie the braid off when you reach a point roughly above the ear.

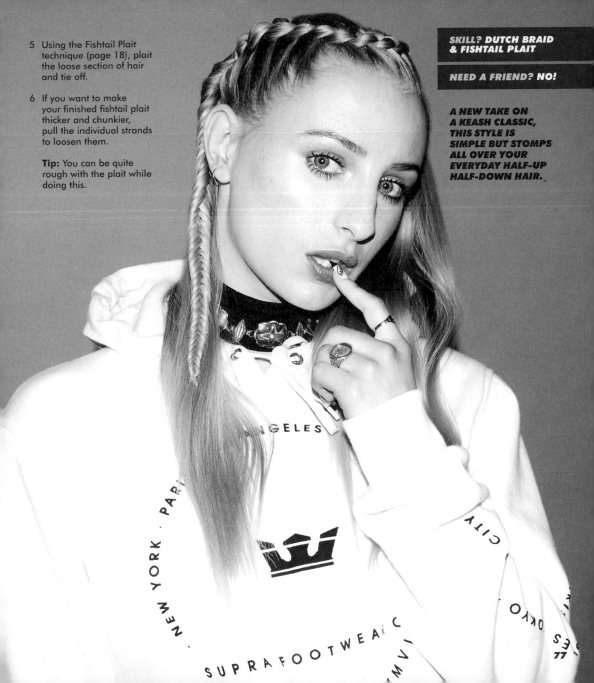

5 Using the Fishtail Plait technique (page 18), plait the loose section of hair and tie off.

6 If you want to make your finished fishtail plait thicker and chunkier, pull the individual strands to loosen them.

Tip: You can be quite rough with the plait while doing this.

A NEW TAKE ON A KEASH CLASSIC, THIS STYLE IS SIMPLE BUT STOMPS ALL OVER YOUR EVERYDAY HALF-UP HALF-DOWN HAIR.

HOOCHIE MAMI

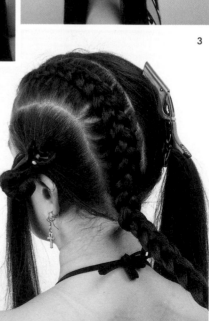

Step-by-step:

1   Begin with a side parting, continuing to the nape of the neck as shown in picture 1, and tie off the smaller section of hair. Now, split the opposite side of hair into two and tie off as shown in pictures 1a and 1b.

2   Let down the smaller section of hair and divide into two sections, starting at the hairline and finishing at the nape of the neck. Clip the lower section out of the way.

3   Braid the upper section front-to-back, to the nape of the neck using the Dutch Braid technique (page 16). Continue with a plait and tie off.

Continued overleaf

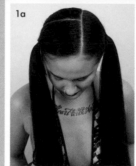

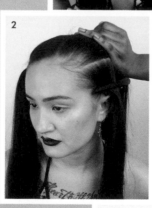

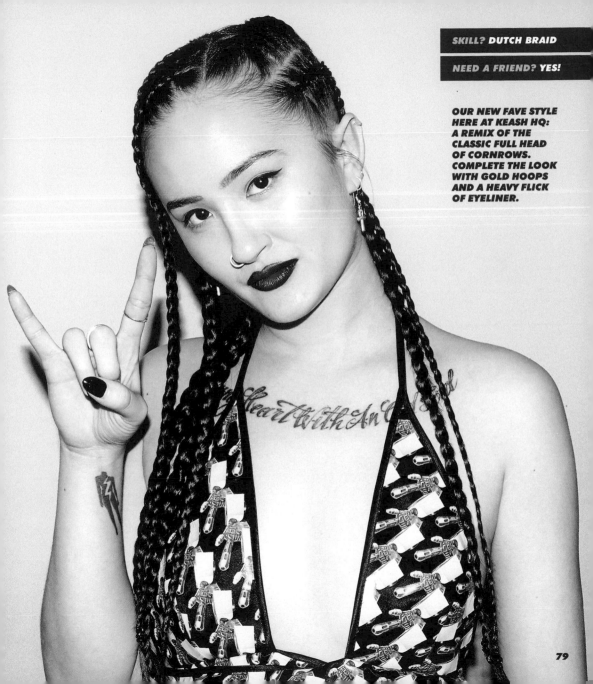

SKILL? DUTCH BRAID

NEED A FRIEND? YES!

OUR NEW FAVE STYLE HERE AT KEASH HQ: A REMIX OF THE CLASSIC FULL HEAD OF CORNROWS. COMPLETE THE LOOK WITH GOLD HOOPS AND A HEAVY FLICK OF EYELINER.

4 Now, unclip the lower section and repeat step 3.

5 Untie the section of hair closest to the face and split into two sections.

6 Again, braid both sections using the Dutch Braid technique (page 16), and continue with plaits to the ends of the hair. The section closest to the face should follow the hairline (framing the face) and sit in front of the ear.

7 Let down the remaining section and again split into two sections as before.

8 Braid both sections to the nape of the neck. Continue with plaits to the ends of the hair and tie off.

4

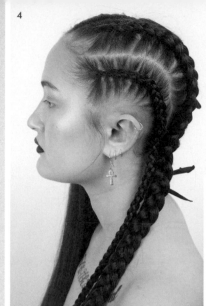

5

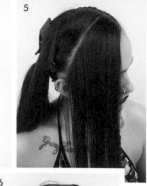

6

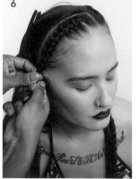

7

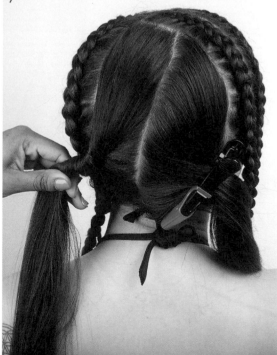

8

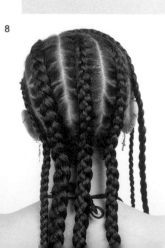

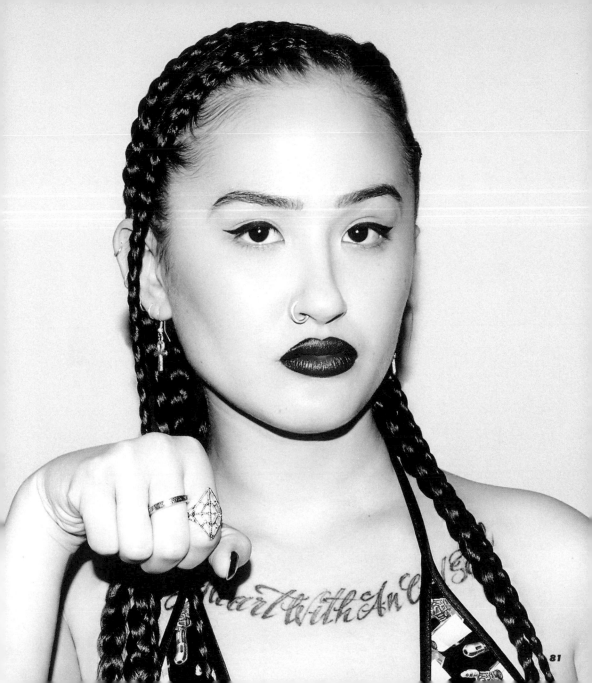

WAVY PONY

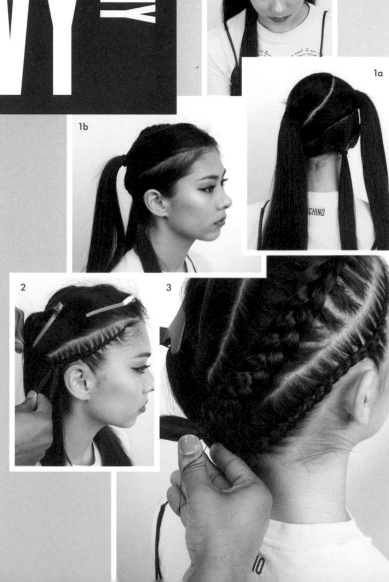

1

1a

1b

Step-by-step:

1 Part the hair into three sections as follows: start with a diagonal parting as shown in picture 1. When you reach the middle of the head, curve the parting around and continue down to the nape of the neck, creating a half-circle shape. Tie off this section. Now, part the remaining hair into two sections and tie off as shown in pictures 1a and 1b.

2 Let down the smallest section of hair above the ear and braid front-to-back using the Dutch Braid technique (page 16). Tie off at the nape of the neck.

   Tip: Use sectioning clips to keep the neighbouring section of hair out of the way.

3 Now, let down and braid, the neighbouring section of hair and tie off at the nape of the neck.

   Continued overleaf

2

3

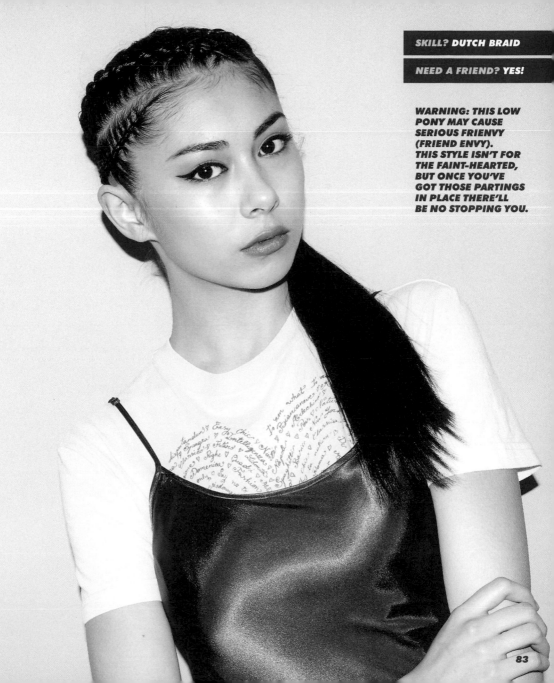

NEED A FRIEND? **YES!**

WARNING: THIS LOW PONY MAY CAUSE SERIOUS FRIENVY (FRIEND ENVY). THIS STYLE ISN'T FOR THE FAINT-HEARTED, BUT ONCE YOU'VE GOT THOSE PARTINGS IN PLACE THERE'LL BE NO STOPPING YOU.

4 Untie the final section
   of hair and create a small
   triangular section with a
   diagonal parting. Clip the
   loose hair back to keep
   out of the way.

5 Braid the new triangular
   section back-to-front,
   using the same Dutch
   Braid technique (page
   16), as before.

6 Once you've braided this
   small section, unclip the
   hair and curve the braid
   down towards the ear.

7 Continue braiding to
   the nape of the neck
   and tie off.

8 Finish the style by tying
   all three braids together
   into a low ponytail.

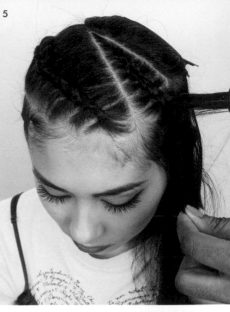

5

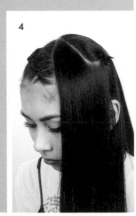

4

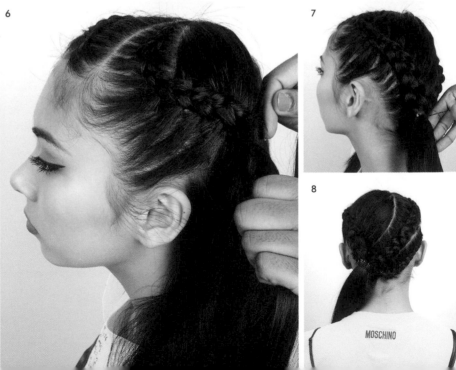

6

7

8

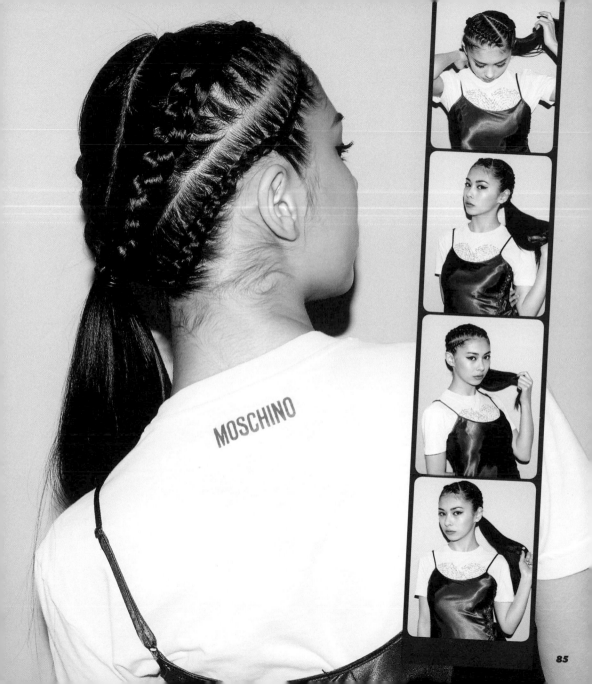

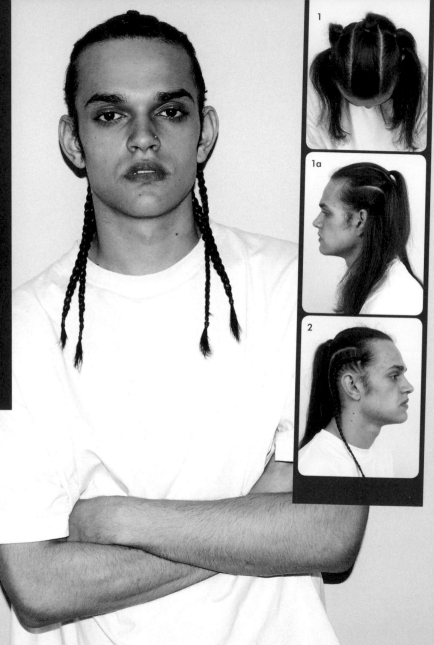

BOY BRAIDS

PT. 2

1

1a

2

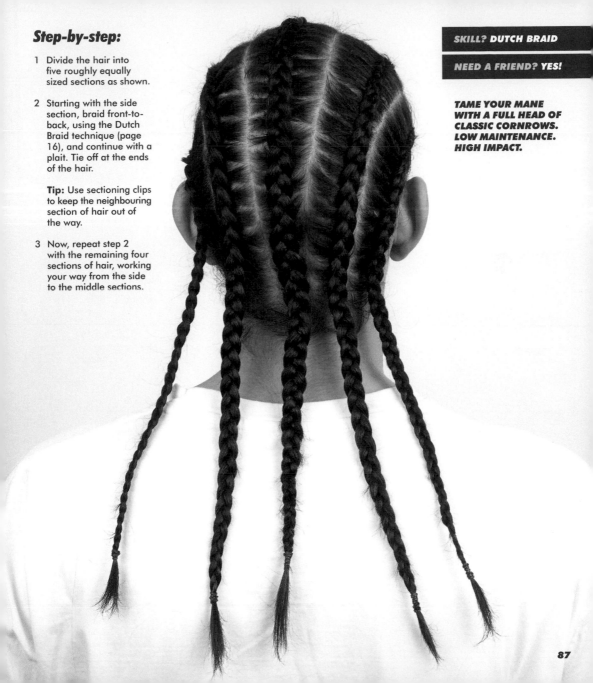

Step-by-step:

1 Divide the hair into five roughly equally sized sections as shown.

2 Starting with the side section, braid front-to-back, using the Dutch Braid technique (page 16), and continue with a plait. Tie off at the ends of the hair.

   Tip: Use sectioning clips to keep the neighbouring section of hair out of the way.

3 Now, repeat step 2 with the remaining four sections of hair, working your way from the side to the middle sections.

SKILL? DUTCH BRAID

NEED A FRIEND? YES!

TAME YOUR MANE WITH A FULL HEAD OF CLASSIC CORNROWS. LOW MAINTENANCE. HIGH IMPACT.

EXTRAS...

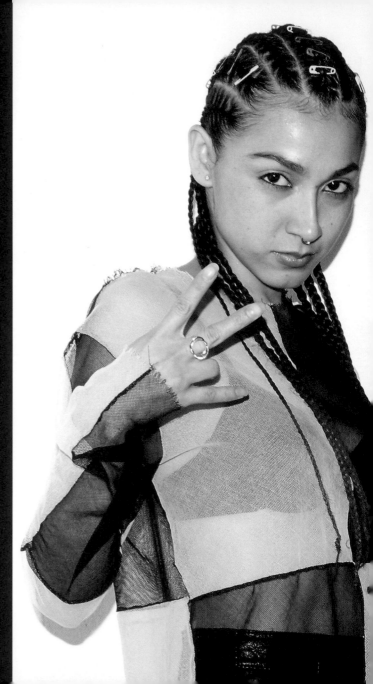

IT'S ALL OR NOTHING
NOW. YOU'VE MADE IT
THIS FAR SO THERE'S NO
POINT HOLDING BACK.
WHETHER YOU WANT
TO ADORN YOUR BRAIDS
WITH JEWELLERY OR
PERSONALISE YOUR
STYLE WITH KISS CURLS,
THIS SECTION IS FOR
THOSE WHO AREN'T
AFRAID TO STAND OUT
FROM THE CROWD.

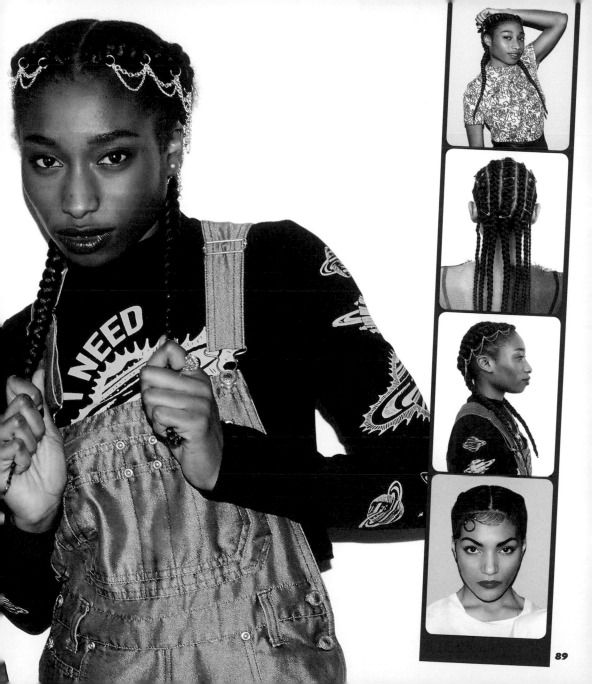

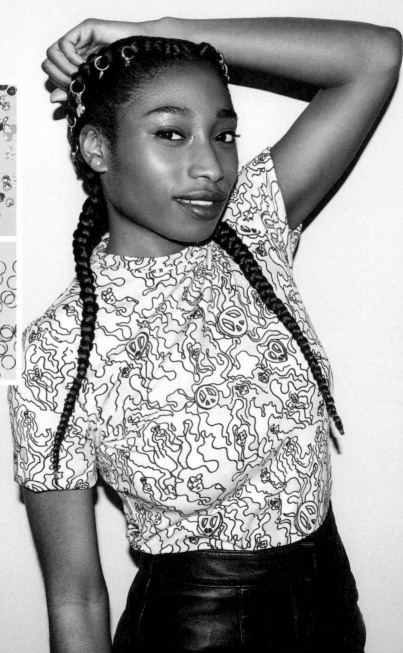

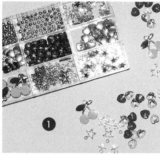

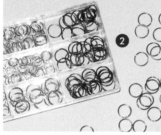

Rings & Charms... Kit:

To add piercings to your plaits, make a pit stop at your nearest bead or craft shop (or go online) and stock up on these essentials to bling up those braids. We use jump rings for hair rings and jewellery charms in a variety of sizes and colours.

1 Hair Charms
2 Hair Rings

90

RINGS & CHARMS

ADDING HAIR RINGS AND CHARMS TO YOUR STYLE IS SUPER QUICK AND EASY... THE HARDEST PART IS DECIDING WHICH CHARMS TO WEAR!

Step-by-step:

1 Choose a selection of hair rings and charms.

   Note: If you don't like adorning your hair with charms, rings work just as great on their own.

2 Prize open a hair ring using your hands and hook a charm onto the ring.

3 Loop the hair ring (with charm) through a strand of the braid.

4 Squeeze the ring shut so the ring and charm is secured to the braid.

5 Keep adding rings and charms until you're happy!

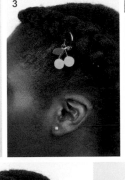

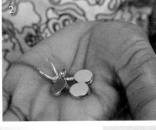

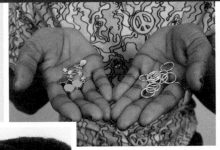

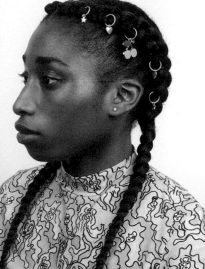

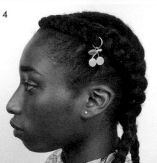

Punk Braids Kit:

Here's the lowdown on hair hardware. You'll find safety pins in most stationery or haberdashery shops, but if you want to up the ante with a variety of sizes and colours then check out your local craft shop or go online (we get ours from eBay). Chains are sold by length in most craft shops and anywhere that supplies jewellery findings, or again, you can head online. For this how-to we've used two sizes of chain (2 mm and 6 mm).

1   Hair Rings
2   Safety Pins
3   Chains

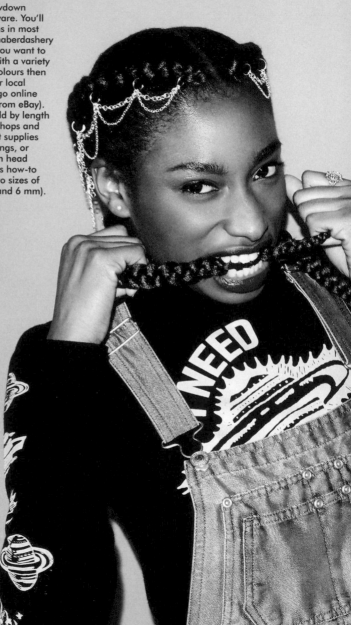

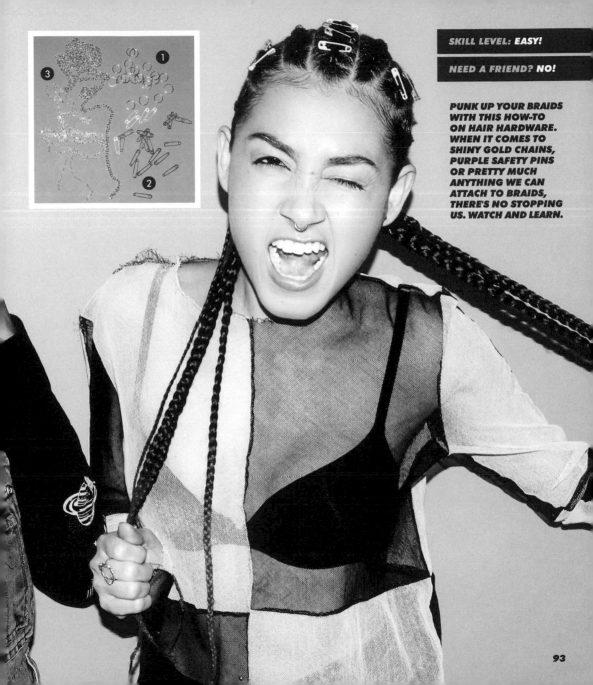

PUNK UP YOUR BRAIDS WITH THIS HOW-TO ON HAIR HARDWARE. WHEN IT COMES TO SHINY GOLD CHAINS, PURPLE SAFETY PINS OR PRETTY MUCH ANYTHING WE CAN ATTACH TO BRAIDS, THERE'S NO STOPPING US. WATCH AND LEARN.

93

Step-by-step:

1 Get yourself a selection of safety pins to add to your braids. We went with coloured safety pins but silver and gold ones look great too!

2 Open the safety pin and slide the pin through the braid.

   Tip: Use a mirror to see what you're doing and be careful when attaching the safety pins.

3 Close the safety pin to secure to the braid.

4 Keep adding safety pins where you want them!

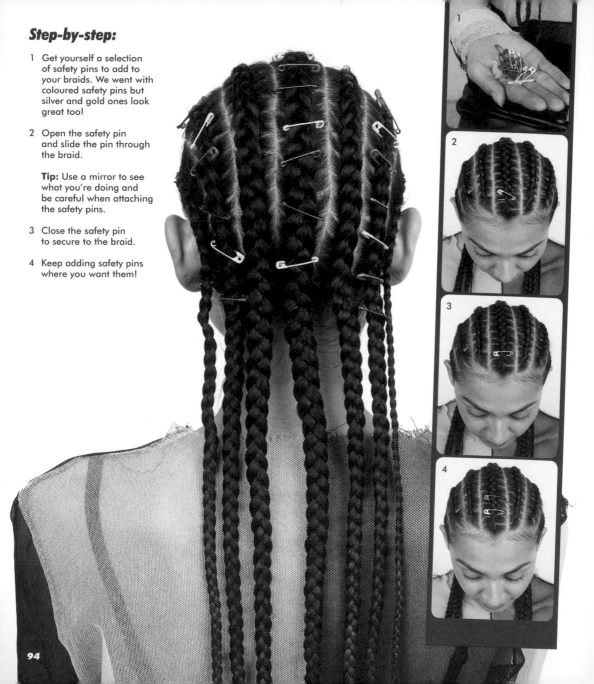

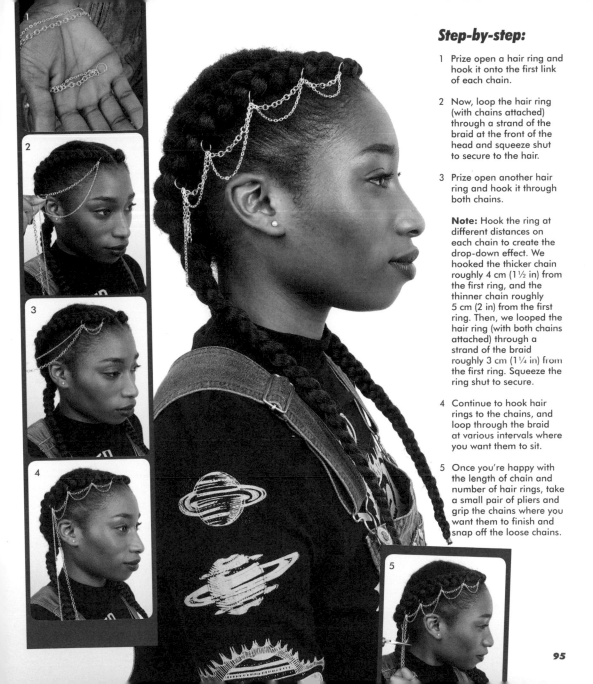

Step-by-step:

1 Prize open a hair ring and hook it onto the first link of each chain.

2 Now, loop the hair ring (with chains attached) through a strand of the braid at the front of the head and squeeze shut to secure to the hair.

3 Prize open another hair ring and hook it through both chains.

   Note: Hook the ring at different distances on each chain to create the drop-down effect. We hooked the thicker chain roughly 4 cm (1½ in) from the first ring, and the thinner chain roughly 5 cm (2 in) from the first ring. Then, we looped the hair ring (with both chains attached) through a strand of the braid roughly 3 cm (1¼ in) from the first ring. Squeeze the ring shut to secure.

4 Continue to hook hair rings to the chains, and loop through the braid at various intervals where you want them to sit.

5 Once you're happy with the length of chain and number of hair rings, take a small pair of pliers and grip the chains where you want them to finish and snap off the loose chains.

KISS CURLS

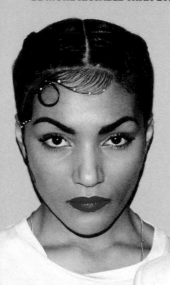
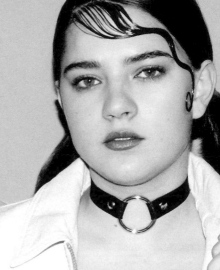

SKILL LEVEL: EASY

NEED A FRIEND? NO!

96

Step-by-step:

1 Take a very small section of hair from the hairline – the more baby hair the better! Style or tie back the rest of the hair to keep out of the way.

2 Dampen the section of hair with a small amount of water (this will prevent the hair gel from drying too quickly). Squeeze a generous amount of gel onto the back of your hand and begin by applying it to the roots with a toothbrush, brushing the hair down flat to your head.

3 Using the toothbrush start to shape your first curl, continuing to flatten the hair to your head.

4 Adding gel as you go, use a pintail comb to curve the hair round to create a wave.

5 Hold the hair in place and create a curve. Keep adding gel to make sure the hair sticks securely to the head.

6 Continue to create waves with the hair until you reach the end of the section. If the kiss curls don't feel secure, top them up with a bit more gel for durability. You can create as many or few curls as you like.

Tip: Once dry, dress-up your kiss curls with gems and diamantes! Use eyelash glue to apply.

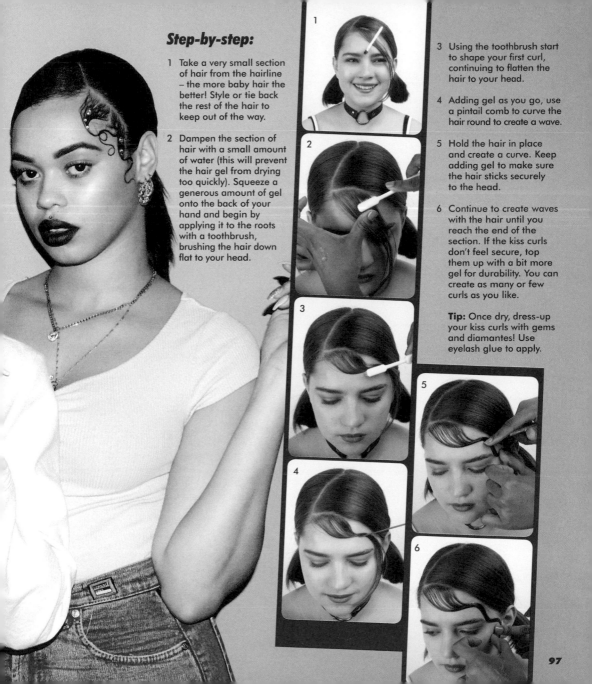

97

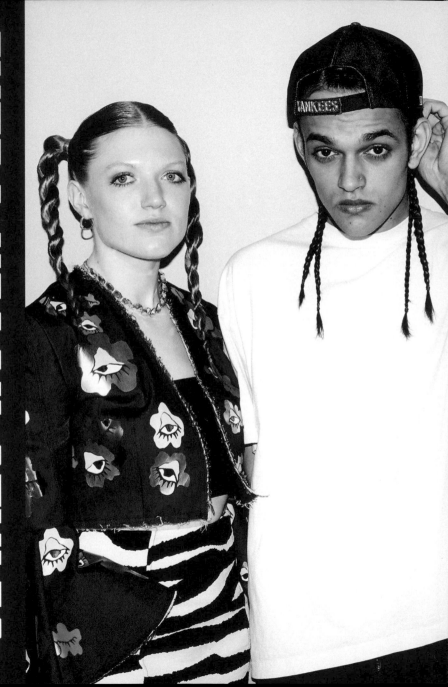

EXTRA KEASH STYLES

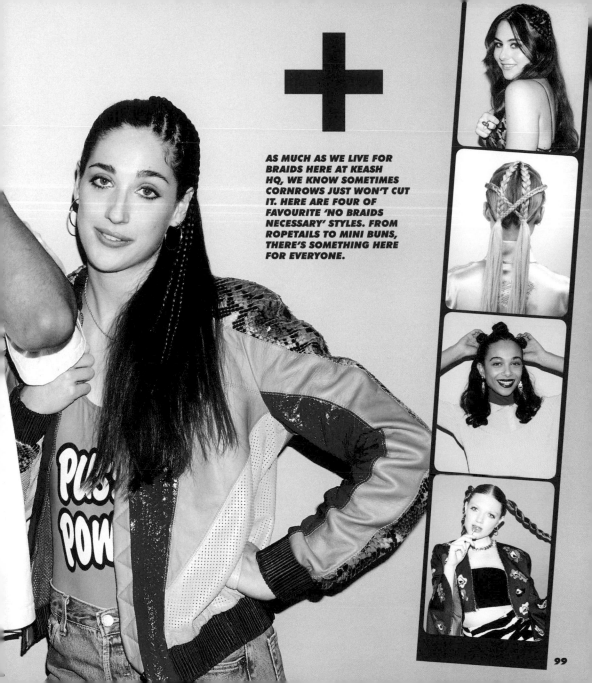

AS MUCH AS WE LIVE FOR BRAIDS HERE AT KEASH HQ, WE KNOW SOMETIMES CORNROWS JUST WON'T CUT IT. HERE ARE FOUR OF FAVOURITE 'NO BRAIDS NECESSARY' STYLES. FROM ROPETAILS TO MINI BUNS, THERE'S SOMETHING HERE FOR EVERYONE.

THE HEART

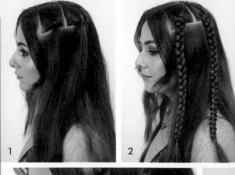

1

2

3

Step-by-step:

1 Begin with a centre parting – be as neat or scruffy as you like! Create two even sections of hair thick enough to create substantial plaits and tie off into ponytails.

2 Plait both ponytails and tie off at the ends temporarily. Now, carefully snip and remove the bands used to tie the initial two plaits.

3 Bulk up your plaits by pulling at the individual strands to make them chunkier.

4 Take the plait closest to the face and twist it around anti-clockwise once (or twice – depending on your hair length) as if you are creating a bun. Secure with a hair grip. Take the remaining plait and twist around clockwise, then secure with a hair grip.

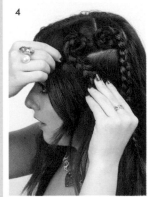

4

5

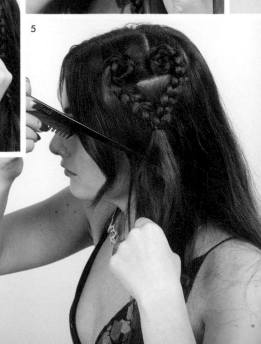

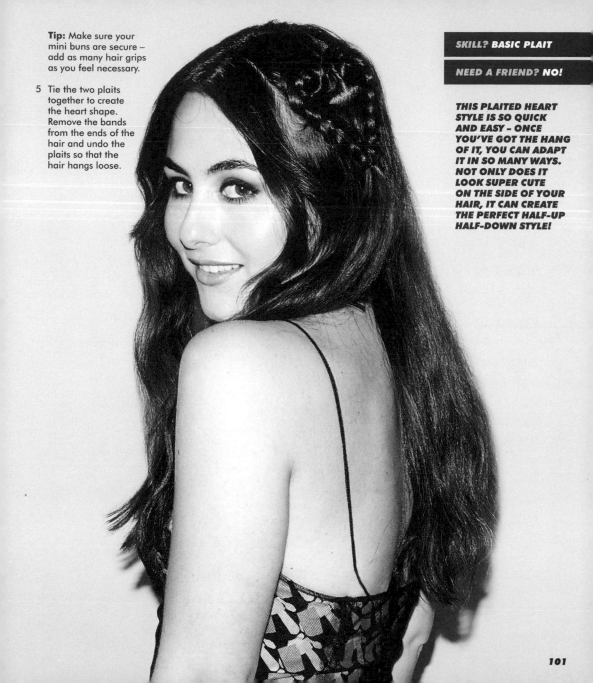

Tip: Make sure your mini buns are secure – add as many hair grips as you feel necessary.

5 Tie the two plaits together to create the heart shape. Remove the bands from the ends of the hair and undo the plaits so that the hair hangs loose.

THIS PLAITED HEART STYLE IS SO QUICK AND EASY – ONCE YOU'VE GOT THE HANG OF IT, YOU CAN ADAPT IT IN SO MANY WAYS. NOT ONLY DOES IT LOOK SUPER CUTE ON THE SIDE OF YOUR HAIR, IT CAN CREATE THE PERFECT HALF-UP HALF-DOWN STYLE!

TWISTED BUNCHES

SKILL? NO BRAIDS

NEED A FRIEND? NO!

YOU'RE NEVER TOO OLD FOR BUNCHES! THIS IS OUR TWISTED TAKE ON BABY-FACED SCHOOLGIRL BRITNEY. ADD FLUFFY HAIR TIES FOR THE FULL EFFECT.

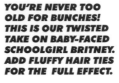

1

2

3

4

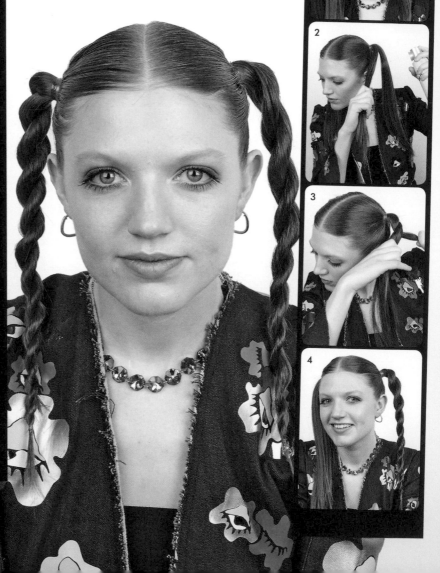

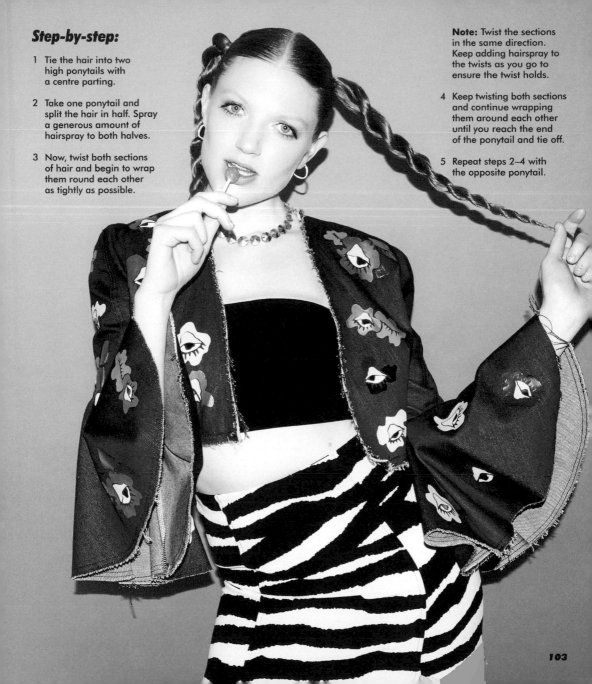

Step-by-step:

1 Tie the hair into two high ponytails with a centre parting.

2 Take one ponytail and split the hair in half. Spray a generous amount of hairspray to both halves.

3 Now, twist both sections of hair and begin to wrap them round each other as tightly as possible.

Note: Twist the sections in the same direction. Keep adding hairspray to the twists as you go to ensure the twist holds.

4 Keep twisting both sections and continue wrapping them around each other until you reach the end of the ponytail and tie off.

5 Repeat steps 2–4 with the opposite ponytail.

THE STAR

SKILL? **BASIC PLAIT**

NEED A FRIEND? **YES!**

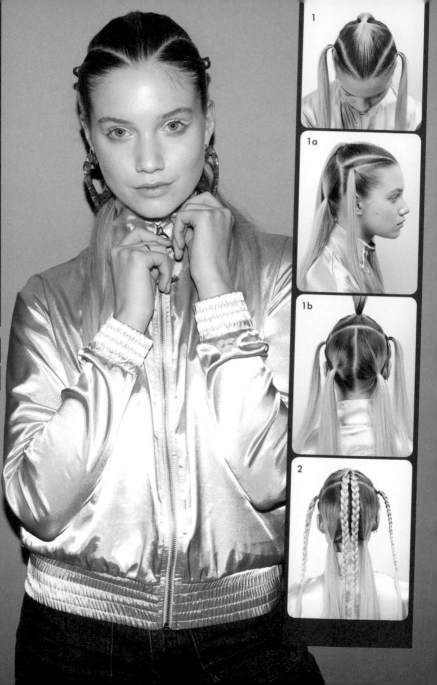

1

1a

1b

2

Step-by-step:

1 Split the hair into five sections as shown in pictures 1–1b. Tie each section tightly into neat and tidy ponytails.

   Note: Be as neat as possible with the partings to create a slick finish.

2 Split the middle ponytail into two and plait both halves. Now, plait the ponytails on either side of the head and tie off all four plaits.

3 Now, start to form the star. Using the plaits from the middle ponytail, tie the left plait to the bottom left ponytail and the right plait to the bottom right ponytail.

4 Next, tie the plait from the left side of the head to the bottom right ponytail.

5 Then tie the plait from the right side of the head to the bottom left ponytail.

6 Remove the hair ties from the loose plaits and brush them out to create two loose ponytails.

INSPIRED BY OUR REBEL POP PRINCESS AND KEASH QUEEN BROOKE CANDY. MIX IT UP BY USING COLOURFUL HAIR TIES OR HAIR BOBBLES.

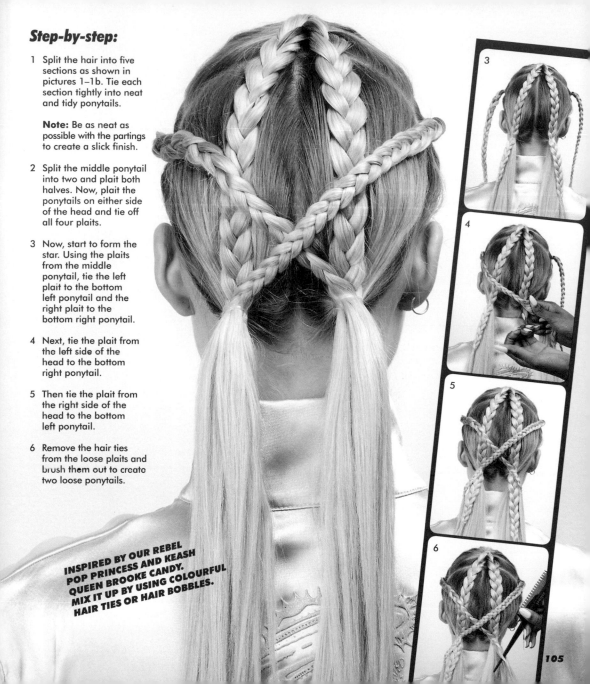

105

BAD GAL BUNS

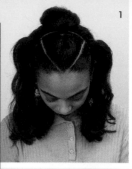

Step-by-step:

1 Part the front section of hair into three sections and tie them into individual ponytails as shown in pictures 1 and 1a. Make sure they are tied neat and tight.

   Note: The sections should look like three triangles.

2 Take one ponytail and twist the loose hair.

3 Once you've twisted the whole ponytail begin to wrap the hair around to create a bun. Finish and secure the bun using a hair grip.

   Tip: Neatly add bands and extra hair grips if the buns don't feel secure.

4 Repeat steps 2–3 with the remaining two ponytails.

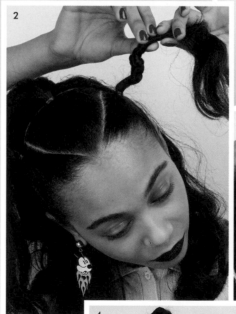

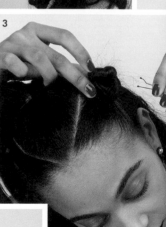

MAKE SPACE BUNS LESS '90S AND MORE NOW BY CHANNELLING YOUR INNER BAD GAL RIRI WITH THIS QUICK AND EASY STYLE. NO BRAIDS NECESSARY!

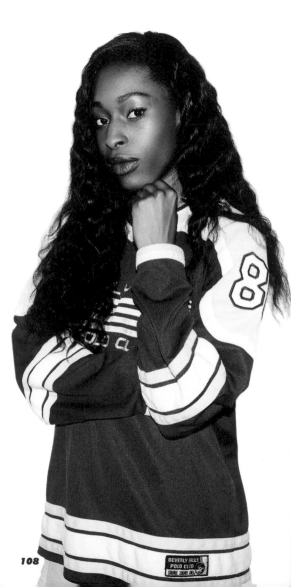

Birthday?
5th November 1989.

Education?
Film Studies and Fashion Styling.

Grew up in...
Kingston, Surrey.

What inspires you to get our of bed in the morning?
Peanut butter on toast – but it has to be crunchy!

What one beauty product could you not live without?
Eyebrow pencil! I cannot imagine what life was like before I started using it.

Describe your style in three words.
Unrefined, baggy, youthful. I know it doesn't sound great but I still look cute... I hope!

Who takes the longest to get ready when you're going out?
Guilty! Unless I have just purchased a new outfit, I have to admit getting dressed is a long-winded process. I have a bad reputation for turning up late because I'm super slow. When I finally get ready, I'm always the one who looks the least dressed up!

What is your wardrobe staple?
A big white T-shirt.

What is your favourite fast food cuisine?
McDonald's for life! I have been trying to plan à McDonald's party for months now but no one's got back to me yet.

Do you plan your daily outfits or do you decide when it's time to get ready?
I like to roughly plan outfits in my head so I can snooze for longer.

Three things on your bucket list?
Horseback ride on the beach, invent something and meet Morgan Freeman.

What environment do you like to work in?
I like to work in an empty silent room. I get distracted so easily and if I play music I just end up dancing around.

Would you rather go on a road trip or lay on a beach for a month?
Road trip around America for sure. I have these vivid images in my mind, all of which I have taken from films.

What advice would you give your younger self?
Love yourself.

Top three styles from the book?
Hoochie Mami (page 78), Double Dutch (page 36) and Wavy Braids (page 40).

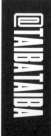

@TAIBATAIBA

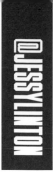

@JESSYLINTON

Do you plan your daily outfits or do you decide when it's time to get ready?
Never pre-plan outfits and always regret it when I have five minutes to leave the house.

Three things on your bucket list?
Live in a different city, write a book – I guess I've ticked that one off?! Party with Rihanna.

What environment do you like to work in?
I work best in my studio. Headphones in, listening to the same album over and over again.

Would you rather go on a road trip or lay on a beach for a month?
Roaaad trip! Reenact scenes from loads of movies.

What advice would you give your younger self?
Don't sweat the small stuff.

Top three styles from the book?
Go Faster Girl (page 32), Hella High Pony (page 78) and Double Dutch (page 36).

Birthday?
16th May 1990.

Education?
Fashion Degree.

Grew up in...
Various parts of suburban South West London.

What inspires you to get our of bed in the morning?
A cup of tea.

What one beauty product could you not live without?
Tinted lip balm. I always have at least two on me.

Describe your style in three words.
Eclectic? Usually quite grungy... and oversized. My mum forever berates me for dressing like a student.

Who takes the longest to get ready when you're going out?
Taiba! We're both always late to the party.

What is your wardrobe staple?
Big baggy sweatshirt.

What is your favourite fast food cuisine?
Pizza!

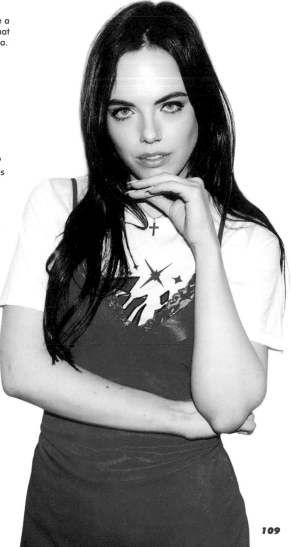

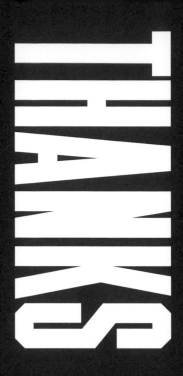

THANKS

Shout out to our awesome braiders and hairstylists Merowe Davis, Amy Purdon, Zateesha Barbour, Freddie Leubner and Claire Moore for helping us to create all the hairstyles in this book.

We are extremely grateful to Kajal Mistry and the team at Hardie Grant for believing in us and to Claire Warner for bringing our vision to life.

Huge thanks to Olivia Richardson for shooting this project and to the rest of the production team Thomas Ramshaw, Phoebe Walters, Trudy Barry, Izabelle Bellamy and Pria Bhamra from Imarni Nails.

For all your generosity and support, many thanks to Palmers, Tangle Teezer, Corioliss, Conair Group, Scünci, ASOS, In Your Dreams, Impossible Project, Jiwinia, Lamoda, Illustrated People, Aries, Unif, Rokit Vintage, Fyodor Golan, Majestic Athletic, This is a Love Song, This Is Welcome, Alternative, Local Heroes, Rascals, Mary Benson, Supra and Jakke.

And finally, thank you to all of our hot mates for modelling for us: Nellie Eden, Laura Ward, Leon Ward, Shannon Mahanty, Jo Saich, Ellie Mercer, Cheyenne Davide, Jada Simone, Yumi Carter, Lucy Shenton, Viviana Gomez, Zara Pearson, Stephanie Tiwo, Morgan Benjamin, Emma Sinclair, Tessa Lawr, Saiara Anwar, Naomi Richardson, Siedah Waller, Robbie Crace, Miranda Chance, Lois Tallulah, Jess Young, Katy Young, Evie Eden, Sophie Sallai, Charlotte Smith and Pippa Christian.

A second thank you to Nellie Eden, not only for modelling, but for writing up the introduction and about our brand.

One final shout out to Raphaelle Moore and Rose Tobin for being Keash groupies from the start.

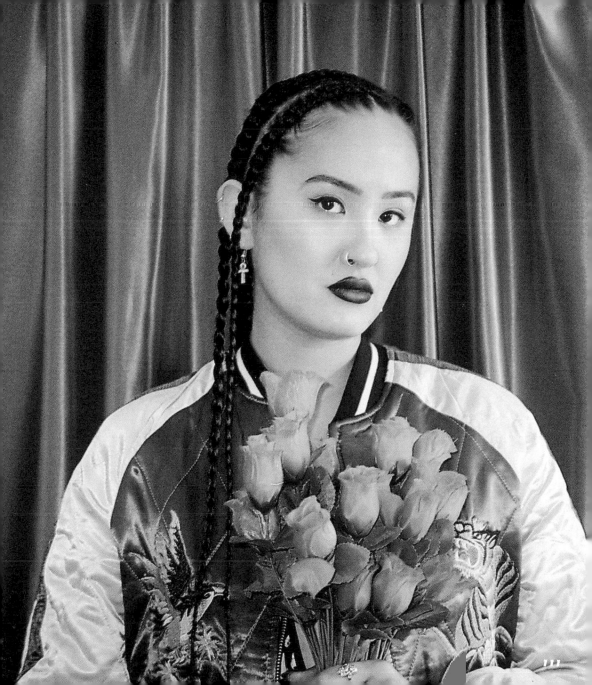

Braid It! by Jessy Linton and Taiba Akhuetie

First published in 2016 by Hardie Grant Books

Hardie Grant Books (UK)
52–54 Southwark Street
London SE1 1UN
hardiegrant.co.uk

Hardie Grant Books (Australia)
Ground Floor, Building 1
658 Church Street
Melbourne, VIC 3121
hardiegrant.com.au

The moral rights of Jessy Linton and Taiba
Akhuetie to be identified as the authors
of this work have been asserted by them
in accordance with the Copyright, Designs
and Patents Act 1988.

Text © Jessy Linton and Taiba Akhuetie
Photography © Olivia Richardson

All rights reserved. No part of this publication
may be reproduced, stored in a retrieval
system or transmitted in any form by any
means, electronic, electrostatic, magnetic
tape, mechanical, photocopying, recording
or otherwise, without the prior written
permission of the Publisher.

British Library Cataloguing-in-Publication
Data. A catalogue record for this book
is available from the British Library.

ISBN: 978-1-78488-053-8

Publisher: Kate Pollard
Commissioning Editor: Kajal Mistry
Editorial Assistant: Hannah Roberts
Cover and Internal Design:
Claire Warner Studio
Photography: Olivia Richardson
Styling: Thomas Ramshaw
Hair: Taiba Akhuetie, Jessy Linton, Merowe
Davis, Amy Purdon, Zateesha Barbour,
Freddie Leubner and Claire Moore
Make-up: Phoebe Walters
Backstage photography: Trudy Barry
Nails: Pria Bhamra (Imarni Nails)
and Izabelle Bellamy

Colour Reproduction by p2d
Printed and bound in China by 1010

10 9 8 7 6 5 4 3 2 1

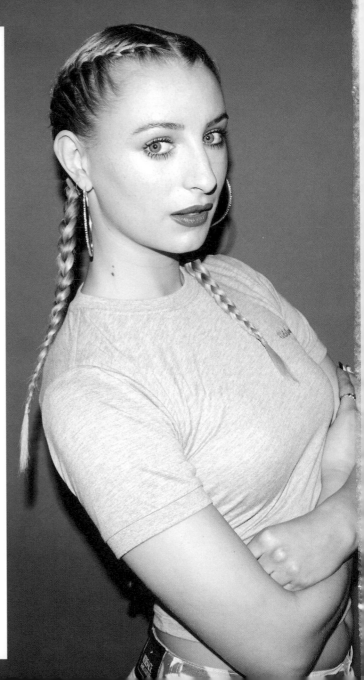

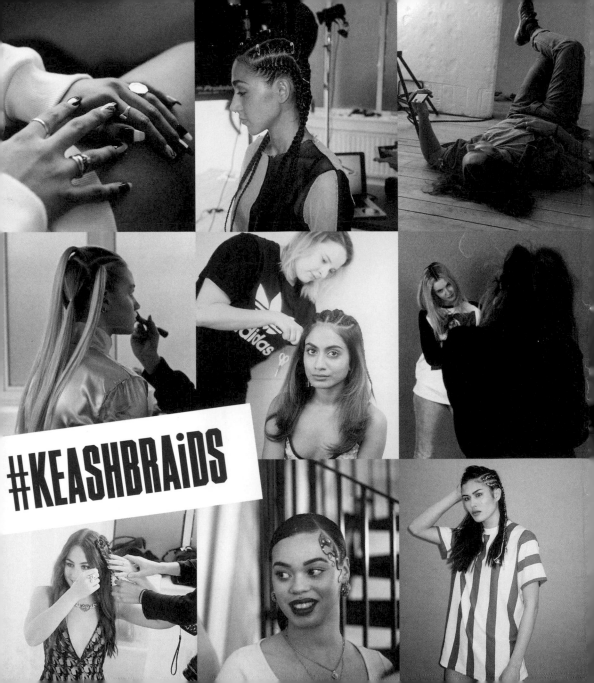

#KEASHBRAiDS